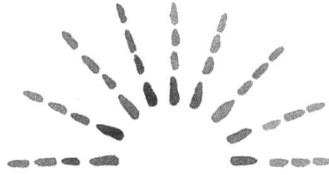

Testimonials

"*After having a baby in my 40s, my usual coping skills and self-care tips really floundered. I realized that my brain would not shut off with a never-ending list of things that I needed to, had to, should do, and all with a load of guilt about how I was failing. My inner self-talk started when I first opened my eyes and actually continued throughout the night with nightmares and lists of work to be completed. I was exhausted, depressed, and defeated. When I took my first dose of stimulants my brain quieted, and I was able to drink a cup of tea and look at my garden without my inner chatter and just be. It brought me to tears.*"

—Mother, Naturopathic Doctor

"*I went through one therapist who I had for three years, two doctors, and one psychiatrist before I found Maggie's care. ADHD had wreaked havoc in my life, but I had figured out a way, as many women do, to mask my symptoms pretty well . . . until I had my first baby. Because these practitioners weren't as well-versed in ADHD as Maggie, it was hard for them to* recognize my host of unique symptoms as ADHD or neurodivergent. Once I found Maggie's care, I felt like I could breathe. Maggie shared so much information about ADHD with me right in the beginning; she would take the time to tell me about her recent findings about ways to help ADHD, or the nervous system, or book recommendations (it seems as if this woman never stops learning). She was the care I didn't know I needed, and she made it possible for me to find the confidence to change my own life."

—Mother with Postpartum Anxiety

"My life has improved so much since being under Maggie's care! For a long time, I had a prescriber who only gave me a script at the end of each appointment but didn't offer any actual support. But I immediately knew that Maggie was different. From the first appointment, she had so much information prepared and had a whole plan for next steps. I went in expecting someone to just give me a script, but instead she listened to me, gave me advice, and helped me finally get on the right balance of meds. I trust Maggie, and I think that is one of the most important things with a health-care provider, especially with mental health. I can confidently say that I've never been happier."

—College Graduate

"I've had difficulty accepting that my struggles were really from ADHD. Maggie helped me work through that difficulty and patiently worked with me as I tried many different kinds of treatments. This eventually made a better daily life for myself and for the patients I helped with the same challenges, too. I've learned a lot from her, both in terms of ADHD-specific treatment knowledge and compassionate care that I am glad to pass on to others. Thank you!"

—Father, Psychiatric Nurse Practitioner

"Maggie's expertise and compassion have been invaluable to me. They've opened a whole new world of information and ongoing research to help us understand ADHD. Her desire for people/patients to understand the legitimacy of the diagnosis has always been genuine. By educating us about the many aspects of ADHD, we've learned a whole new template for self-evaluation, and awareness of the negative self-talk and blame that had taken root. Maggie advocates for us and helps us advocate for ourselves!"

—Hospital Social Worker

"Before being treated for ADHD, I saw myself in a very isolated way. I felt alone. I viewed my inability to bring tasks to completion as there being something 'wrong' with me. I saw the scattered-ness of my brain and the actions that followed as being a 'bad' thing. After being treated, I still think there's something 'different' about me, but it doesn't carry a negative connotation. Because of Maggie's compassion and honesty, I have changed my mind set about my differences and no longer equate being different with something negative. It's just different. I have realized that I am far from being alone in these feelings, and that's comforting. Having a therapist like Maggie who is straightforward and 'tuned in' is imperative in *the process of feeling better about yourself. When you know someone is really listening and your voice is being heard, it's amazing how much you can accomplish."*

—Bodybuilder, Grandmother

"Before being treated, I spent a lot of time ruminating over priorities, deadlines, and how to manage my schedule. I was consumed by imposter syndrome and was convinced my colleagues would see right through my act; I replayed even the most minor mistakes in my head continuously, feeling embarrassment days (weeks, months, even years) after the 'mistake' occurred. After being treated, I implemented a number of the suggestions Maggie offered: reviewing priorities with my manager weekly, setting realistic deadlines for myself, and letting others know if an expectation was not realistic. My output has improved, as well as my feelings of accomplishment. The imposter syndrome and negative self-talk still occur, but they aren't as debilitating as before. I hope in sharing my own mistakes I can help others embrace theirs as well."

—Business Manager

"For much of my life, I believed a ceaseless cycle of procrastination, distraction, accompanying anxiety, and frustration to be a prerequisite of every task, typical of the lived experience of every human being. It wasn't until late in high school, while doing homework one afternoon with my best friend, that I noticed she did not have the same task-initiating woes I did.

"I was at my wits end, burnt out and depressed by the time I was referred to Maggie by my therapist. I was previously

diagnosed with ADHD by another practitioner but was deterred by an adverse reaction to meds and an overall lack of understanding about what it meant to have an ADHD brain. In the 17-ish months since my initial meeting with Maggie, my prior diagnosis was reaffirmed, and I am much better equipped to be a person with ADHD.

"With genetic testing, Maggie was able to determine what class of meds would be most compatible with my specific ADHD brain; with blood work, she identified my nutrient deficiencies and the supplements I should take to boost them; through the titrating process, she provided guidance on getting to my ideal dosage of methylphenidate.

"Additionally, Maggie's comprehensive explanation of rejection sensitive dysphoria helped me make sense of what I minimized, for a long time, as being irrationally sensitive. For most of my life, I have experienced so much frustration at feeling driven but, conversely, aimless and stuck. Now, I feel like I finally have the tools to shift my drive into gear."

—**Artist & Designer**

"Working with Maggie has had one of the most profound impacts on my life. I had suspicions throughout my life that ADHD might be part of my story, but having been born in the cusp years of Xennials, I did not have the fortitude of cultural support to follow those hunches. Perimenopause finally pushed me into spaces that felt overwhelming with no reprieve. I was trying to be Superwoman and couldn't keep up.

"Thanks to Maggie, I learned that I was a high-functioning ADHDer—having forged a demanding career in commercial real estate while supporting and providing steadfast support to my immediate family. Working with Maggie has opened many doors, immense understanding, and mind-blowing discoveries of what was and has been happening with my brain chemistry and potentially those around me.

"Maggie's passion for this journey is infectious, and her ability to tap into her client's experience is a true example of deep compassion and sincerity. Her insights are powerful, and I attribute the betterment of my life to her since working with her in the last year. My compassion meter is fully activated most of the time, and I find myself in a place of grace with others."

—Business Manager

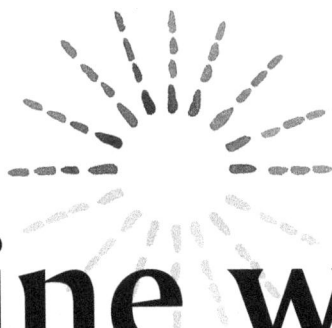

Shine with
ADHD

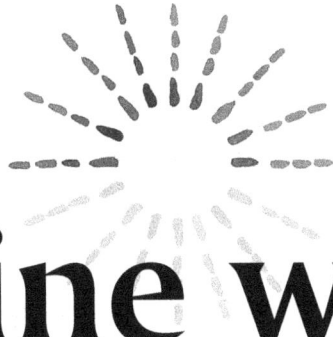

Shine with
ADHD

Unlock Your Potential with Skills, Medicine, and Micronutrients

MAGGIE ALEXANDER, MS, PMHNP

PYP **Publish** Your Purpose

For permission requests, write to the publisher, addressed "Attention: Permissions Coordinator," at the address below.

Publish Your Purpose
141 Weston Street, #155
Hartford, CT, 06141

PYP **Publish** Your Purpose

The opinions expressed by the Author are not necessarily those held by Publish Your Purpose.

Ordering Information: Quantity sales and special discounts are available on quantity purchases by corporations, associations, and others. For details, contact the author at shinewithadhdbook@gmail.com.

Edited by: Connie J. Mayse, Kelsey Spence
Cover design by: Nelly Murariu
Cover Illustration by: Andi Schrader
Author Headshot: Eloika Rozendaal
Typeset by: Medlar Publishing Solutions Pvt Ltd., India

Printed in the United States of America.

ISBN: 979-8-88797-184-1 (hardcover)
ISBN: 979-8-88797-185-8 (paperback)
ISBN: 979-8-88797-186-5 (ebook)

Library of Congress Control Number: 2025911787

First edition, January 2026.

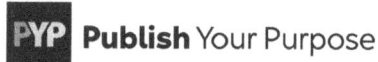

The information contained within this book is strictly for informational purposes. The material may include information, products, or services by third parties. As such, the Author and Publisher do not assume responsibility or liability for any third-party material or opinions. The publisher is not responsible for websites (or their content) that are not owned by the publisher. Readers are advised to do their own due diligence when it comes to making decisions.

Publish Your Purpose is a hybrid publisher of non-fiction books. Our mission is to elevate the voices often excluded from traditional publishing. We intentionally seek out authors and storytellers with diverse backgrounds, life experiences, and unique perspectives to publish books that will make an impact in the world. Do you have a book idea you would like us to consider publishing? Please visit PublishYourPurpose.com for more information.

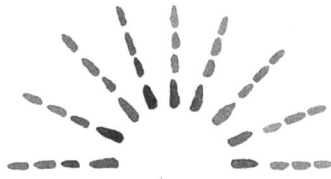

Dedication

My dear clients, you have been my greatest teachers.
You entrusted me with your personal lives
and helped me to learn new approaches and techniques
that deepen the impact of my practice.
Your experience will help to improve thousands of lives.
You are my heroes.

I am so very grateful.

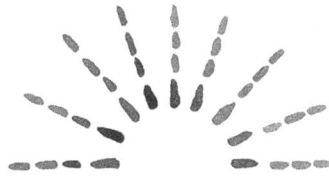

Contents

Contents

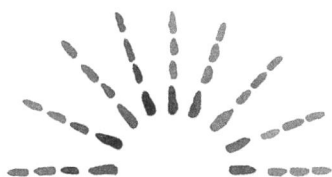

Acknowledgments

Dr. Richard Sogn, in 2013, you opened your office doors to me when I was a brand-new psychiatric nurse practitioner and, with that, enabled me to enter this rewarding work with confidence.

Dr. William Dodson, you have been a mainstay for me and my clients through your tireless efforts to understand ADHD and share your knowledge of the use of stimulants and understanding of rejection sensitivity with the public and health professionals.

Dr. James Greenblatt, you taught about the power of micronutrients, provided functional medicine teachings, and created the professional organization Psychiatry Redefined. Through your work and many books, you have enabled thousands of providers to practice integrative medicine. I use your teachings each and every day; thank you.

Dr. Sandra Kooij, you authored one of the only textbooks on ADHD and conducted vital research on women and how ADHD uniquely affects them. You were an inspiration to me and hundreds of others at the World Congress on ADHD in Amsterdam in 2023; thank you.

Dr. Stephen Faraone, thank you for making your valuable evidence-based research and findings available to ADHD patients and health-care practitioners around the globe.

Institute for Functional Medicine, thank you for allowing me to use some of your work in this book and for making critical root cause information and training easily accessible to providers like me.

Mari Alexander, thank you for introducing me to the reality of ADHD's existence and showing me many of its charms.

Brenda Fox, thank you for your steady support and belief in my commitment to educating others who have not had the opportunities I have and are ready to make better choices.

Joyce Allen, thank you for your expert initial editing and complete confidence in my ability to complete this labor of love.

Connie Mayse, your expertise as a copy editor increased my confidence in sharing this content with my readers and fellow practitioners; thank you ever so much.

Finally, and at the core of my heart, I offer thanks to my children. My deepest hope is that I have helped to make your lives richer and that you know how very much I love you.

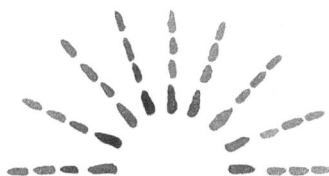

Foreword

This is the book that I wish had been available years and years ago before I treated thousands of patients with ADHD. It is very rare to have writing on a medical condition that is both thorough and accurate but still remains easily accessible to the average person. *Shine with ADHD* achieves both of these goals beautifully: It proves that a scientifically rigorous text can still speak empathically to the souls of people who are in a lifelong struggle to master their own divergent nervous systems. There are few things in life that have a more profound impact than to be fully understood and accepted for who you are.

This book is invaluable in the process of trying to wrap your head around a condition that is unlike any other. For many people, ADHD is a far cry from anything they've dealt with before, whether in medicine, behavioral health, or elsewhere in their lives. Those living with ADHD must have a guide who is not only extremely knowledgeable and fact-based, but also compassionate, wise, and down-to-earth. Without that, realistic and attainable goals too easily get sidetracked, and those with ADHD find themselves back at square one. Unfortunately, due to a lack of national practice guidelines, clinicians have been inadequately trained in how to treat the 10 percent of the population who live with what, for many, is a debilitating condition.

In *Shine with ADHD*, Maggie Alexander explores how ADHD is often a family affair because of the strong contribution of genetics and neurology to every aspect of the condition. If an adult has ADHD, half of their genetic relatives (their parents, siblings, and their children) will also have ADHD. This leaves parents not only having to manage their own ADHD but also raising children of whom at least half will be affected similarly. Parents know that raising children with ADHD is a far different task from raising their other children, and there is often a sense of both urgency and powerlessness in their efforts to make sure that their children do not have to endure what they went through. This book is necessary reading for the entire family, because ADHD affects everyone in the family, and the guidance in these pages is indispensable in setting up a home in which everyone is accepted and supported.

Even more importantly, this book strives to counter the common misunderstanding and disinformation around ADHD, which may be the condition that people have the most misconceptions about. Everyone with ADHD needs to have someone trustworthy and knowledgeable to help them separate the falsehoods from the universally agreed upon facts, especially when so many people in the United States still have the unconscious attitude that the treatment of ADHD has more potential harms than the condition itself. It's a tragedy that so many shy away from doing anything about their ADHD because of the false information they are exposed to. Knowledge is power, and this book is the best "self-defense manual" available. I recommend it to anyone living with ADHD and their clinicians.

In 2026, ADHD is no longer a controversial condition. The original concerns have now been thoroughly studied and managed, but all that life-changing information remains out of the hands of many doctors and their patients. Maggie Alexander distills all of the necessary facts you need and constantly redirects you (and your clinician, as well) toward the best, most reliable resources and insights available from guidelines across the world. She empowers her readers to recognize their unique brain chemistry and educate themselves on the many positive attributes of living with ADHD. Through building consistent skills, finding root causes of common micronutrient deficiencies, and the precise use of medicine, *Shine with ADHD* becomes a powerful tool that enables the person to not only discover new solutions to old problems, but build replicable systems to actualize those new ideas.

Now it's time to get started!

Bill Dodson, MD LF-APA
Expert in the treatment of ADHD
ADDitude Magazine, Medical Review Panel member
Author of 120 articles and 17 webinars for *ADDitude Magazine*, ADD.org
Author, *The Recognition and Treatment of ADHD*, to be published in 2026

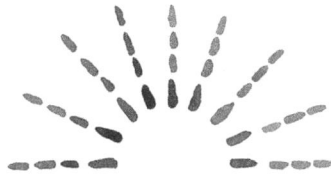

Introduction

Welcome. This book is written for you, the person living with Attention Deficit Hyperactivity Disorder (ADHD). You, who feel creative and clever in one moment and in the next wonder why you just can't get stuff done. You, the person who loves someone who has trouble tracking boring details and yet can hear and see your uniqueness better than most. You, the practitioner who was told to treat depression and anxiety first, or even worse, that ADHD just isn't a thing and that these clients are drug-seeking. I don't have ADHD, and I didn't recognize it in my family members. Even more so, I thought most mental health issues could be addressed with three things: broccoli, love, and exercise. These are three great approaches, but not nearly enough to address the neurotransmitter deficit for those living with ADHD.

Although I share some background information on the characteristics of ADHD, this book is not meant to be a primer. There are other books written about ADHD's incidence and basic treatment protocols. I am sharing the knowledge that I've gained through studying with some of the top ADHD physicians and functional medicine providers in the United States and through working closely with my clients. These beautiful people begin to thrive when they find the precise medication and dose, coupled with helpful micronutrients and learned skills.

I've written this book from the perspective of my 600+ clients who have taught me what ADHD is and isn't. In the pages ahead, I share their stories, current research and clinical practice, medical treatments, and the powerful tools I've learned from functional medicine to address and treat this condition.

Some prefer not to call ADHD a *disorder*, but rather, as Dr. Edward Hallowell says, Variable Attention Stimulus Trait (VAST). As he and Dr. John Ratey aptly describe in their latest book, *ADHD 2.0*, VAST can include great genius and crippling states of procrastination, distraction, and inability to complete tasks.

My hope is that whether you suffer from ADHD or are a provider to or loved one of someone with ADHD, you find so much hope within these pages. You will come to realize, as I did, that the face of ADHD is not just a nine-year-old boy throwing a rock through a window; it is also the dreamy-eyed girl staring out the window. It is the irritable, anxious employee who double-checks their work and spends extra time on weekends to ensure they are doing a good job. It is the depressed college student who does most of the work for their assignment but then oversleeps and doesn't turn it in on time. And yes, it is also that guy who keeps interrupting you and tapping his foot. It can also be one of your top team members who spends time outside of work, going the extra mile and double checking that they aren't letting someone down.

But seeking help is hard, because in addition to these challenging traits, living with ADHD also means you are authentic, able to absorb large amounts of data, have a strong sense of justice, are innovative, and are able to get a huge amount done in a short time. You are also passionate, energetic, enthusiastic, progressive, visionary, and, likely, humble. These aspects are highly desirable, yet they don't help improve your concentration when you have to do a boring task.[1]

I have worked with hundreds of clients who have found greater peace of mind, improved academic or career success, and better relationships with the people who matter most. Some elected to leave ineffective relationships, others went back to school, and still others dared to change jobs or travel. Most have come to know and love themselves far better than before they understood they were living with ADHD and found proper treatment. A fitting analogy is that they could not see well, and they were prescribed glasses. The right prescription afforded them the ability to focus much more clearly, offering them previously unrealized stamina and emotional regulation. You'll find many of their stories scattered throughout this book.

It would be an understatement to say I am thrilled to be a guide on their journeys. I am deeply honored and grateful to all the clients and their families who have entrusted me with their care. You have taught me how to help others realize their dreams.

----

[1] Claire Sehinson, "An Introduction to Neurodiversity in Clinical Practice," PsychiatryRedefined.org (2023): 16, https://www.psychiatryredefined.org/wp-content/uploads/2023/09/Claire-Sehinson-Introduction-to-Neurodiversity-in-Clinical-Practice_Psychiatry-Redefined.pdf.

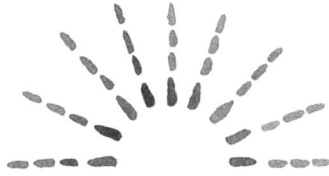

CHAPTER 1

From Nonbeliever to Passionate Advocate—Beyond Broccoli, Love, and Exercise

Before I was treated for ADHD, I was seen by five counselors and four doctors for anxiety and depression. I tried three different antidepressants and was given Xanax and sleeping pills. I lost two jobs. There were times when I was so depressed, I thought about giving up all together. My boyfriend kept telling me I was smart, and my college professors told me I was great in class, but I just couldn't get my papers completed. It took me six years to finish college, and my boyfriend left me because I wasn't paying attention to what he was saying to me. After I got treated and I could focus on more than my love for sports, I started being more productive and I was able to get my first design job that led to the one I have now and really love. My boss tells me I'm one of the most creative people on the team, and I'm learning ways to stay on task and finish projects mostly on time. I feel so much calmer, and I am sleeping better. My depression is gone, and I only feel anxious around deadlines and when I have company over. The one medication I'm on is Adderall. It's so much better. I feel like myself, just focused, and now I know it wasn't just me being a mess-up.

After 25 years of being a nurse-midwife, delivering 1,500 babies, I was convinced that all mental health issues could be addressed with three things: broccoli, love, and exercise. I went back to school to become a psychiatric nurse practitioner in hopes of helping depressed and anxious pregnant women and new mothers. I didn't believe in ADHD and wasn't keen on prescribing lots of antidepressants. Diet, exercise, and therapy seemed like the right therapeutic solution to me.

My life, career, and goals changed soon after I met Matthew (not his real name). Matt, an IT professional in his 40s, married with kids, handsome, and athletic, was sent to see me by his doctor. He'd been depressed and had tried three different anti-depressants, but things kept getting worse. By the time he was referred to me as a brand-new psychiatric nurse practitioner, he was suicidal. I wondered, why was this happily married guy, with a good job and in perfect physical health, suicidal? Clearly, broccoli, love, and exercise had not worked for him, nor had three different antidepressants.

He told me that as a high school junior he began hanging out with the kids who drank and smoked weed. His grades sank from As and Bs to Cs and Ds. Then his dad sent him off to a treatment program. Someone there prescribed him some Adderall, and his father put him in a private high school where they supposedly didn't drink and smoke. Sure enough, he earned straight As his senior year.

I was deeply worried. What could I do for this guy? A switch flipped in my brain. Maybe it wasn't just the private high school, maybe it was the medication, Adderall. Maybe he had a diagnosis I didn't previously believe in: ADHD. I was nervous to prescribe a drug like Adderall, which I wrongly thought was too strong or even addictive. I was still misinformed about its risks. Instead, I gave him a child's dose of Concerta, the extended-release version of Ritalin.

Three days later, Matt phoned. "Hello?" I said, but he was already speaking. "Oh my God, Maggie!" he blurted out. "Remember I told you that in an eight-hour day, I was barely doing an hour of work?"

"Yeah," I replied. "Well, I worked all day yesterday!" He was ecstatic. "Furthermore, remember how I told you I'd be so tired every afternoon that I'd have to take a two-hour nap before dinner?" "Yes, I remember, Matt."

"Not only did I work all day, but I came home and played with my kids!" He was laughing on the phone. "I played with them for an hour, had dinner, and put them to bed just like a normal dad!"

His joy was breathtaking. I choked up. "This is great, Matt," I said, my voice full of emotion. After I hung up, I became very curious.

This was my watershed moment, when a football field of floodlights went off in my head. ADHD exists. It's a real thing. In Matt's case, a tiny dose of Ritalin changed a suicidal man who'd been depressed for over a decade into a productive person who reengaged with his wife and children. It is rewarding to note that Matt and his wife have now successfully coparented for 12 years, and his kids are excelling in school.

The experience with Matt changed the course of my life and practice. I realized that, just as in my own personal experience and that of my clients and family members, there are thousands more who have been let down by the almost universal lack of knowledge about the effective treatment of ADHD.

This is the story of how the right dosage of the right medication, a few micronutrients, and developing a deep understanding of what ADHD is and is not can radically change the lives of those living with ADHD.

Do you have ADHD and feel your life sliding away from you? Are your goals seemingly unachievable? Are you tired of living with the same, hopeless feeling of not living up to your potential? I wrote this book for you, your loved ones, and your care providers. A much better future is possible and is within your grasp.

ADVICE

My greatest teachers have been the clients with ADHD who I've served since 2013. I asked them to share their best advice with you.

Each chapter will include some stories and lessons learned, but I want to give you a burst of inspiration right at the start. Here are some gems from everyday men and women who live with ADHD:

"When I learned that my trouble tracking information, completing tasks on time, and tendency to degrade myself for what I thought was constant disappointment was from my ADHD, I cried. I experienced so much grief and thought

about what might have been if I'd only known sooner. Ultimately, your diagnosis is a blessing. You now have ways to address your pain."

"Feelings of loss are normal, part of the adjustment, and improve with time. Try to be compassionate to yourself; you deserve grace for all you've been through. You are amazing."

"It is a wonderful journey to get to know your true self. You are worth it."

"Prioritize self-love, acceptance, and patience with yourself. Go at your own pace and surround yourself with people who understand, and who you can be open about it with. It is not something to be ashamed of; it will set you free to be able to live a life so much more fulfilling."

"Take the 'onboarding' process slowly and be ready to keep your eyes and mind wide open—it's weird at first. Give yourself a lot of grace. You're expected to struggle. Be open about the experience; it's easier not to do it alone. Ultimately, discover what 'system/regimen' works for you. Know that you'll be stumbling and messing up until you land on the 'right' one. The right one is the one that's easy, 'no brainer,' and it sticks."

"Ask for help, ask for accommodation, work on understanding the areas that you struggle in, and figure out what you need to help you."

"Share what you learn with someone close to you— partner, friend, relative. My biggest epiphanies have come when trying to explain to my husband what I've learned and how it makes me feel."

"Practitioners, if you have not read credible sources of research and legitimate information on ADHD in the last decade, please get curious and educated for the sake of your patients. Be honest with yourself if you have a negative view of the diagnosis, or of people who carry the diagnosis. There are probably assumptions you have made that are incorrect and can be unpacked and thrown away and replaced with some current information."

Each chapter in this book will conclude with a list of "pearls."

CHAPTER 1 PEARLS

1. Your life will improve greatly by educating yourself about ADHD. This is a genetic condition; you and your parents did nothing wrong.

2. The number one treatment for ADHD is medication; the correct drug and dosage matter a great deal.

3. The ideal dosage of medication—Ritalin or Adderall—is not related to your sex, age, or size but is unique to you.

4. Addressing ADHD first may improve, or even eliminate, your depression and anxiety.

5. Sharing your experience with trusted others will help you integrate your newfound learning and help lead you to greater success sooner.

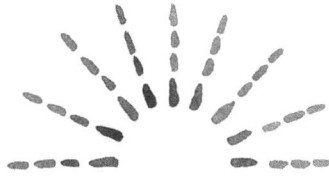

CHAPTER 2

What ADHD Is and Isn't

Not everyone is a "Tigger." Some people's hyperactivity only shows up in their brains.

THE MANY FACES OF ADHD

When my children were in school, they were focused on sports, dance, specialized computer skills, reading, and friends. They were not hyperactive; one was the lead in the school musical, and another made short movies that required hours and hours of focused concentration. I thought they could not possibly have ADHD. However, getting started on boring homework assignments, regulating their sleep schedules, and shutting down their brains from worry seemed especially hard. I fed them broccoli, loved them a lot, and ensured they exercised regularly. It wasn't until after I met Matt that I realized maybe my own teenage children had ADHD!

> **attention deficit hyperactivity disorder (ADHD)**
> A developmental disorder marked by inattention, impulsivity, and/or hyperactivity.

ADHD has been recognized by all the major medical associations that support pediatrics, family medicine, and psychiatry in the United States. These include the American Academy of Pediatrics, the Academy of Family Physicians, the American Medical Association, the American Psychiatric Association, and the National Institute of Health. Unfortunately, due to inadequate medical education, health-care providers and other mental health practitioners are undereducated, and numerous myths prevail when it comes to understanding ADHD. Many professionals, and much of the public population, still believe that ADHD is not actually a real disorder and are unaware that it is due to deficiencies in the person's neurotransmitters. It is still a common belief that if someone doesn't behave in a hyperactive manner or has done reasonably well in school or at work, they cannot have ADHD. Most people are reluctant to use stimulant medications for fear of becoming addicted, and they don't recognize the importance of taking them consistently and at a very precise dose to achieve an optimum level of concentration.

ADHD is one of the most common neurodevelopmental disorders in children and adolescents.[2] The prevalence of ADHD in children and adolescents nationally is 11.4 percent of the population.[3] The prevalence of adult ADHD in the US is 6 percent; internationally (in the Americas, Europe, and Middle East), it is 3.4 percent of the population.[4] It decreases

[2] U.S. Centers for Disease Control and Prevention, "About Attention-Deficit/Hyperactivity Disorder (ADHD)," CDC.gov, October 23, 2024, https://www.cdc.gov/adhd/about/index.html.

[3] U.S. Centers for Disease Control and Prevention, "Data and Statistics on ADHD," CDC.gov, November 19, 2024, https://www.cdc.gov/adhd/data/index.html.

[4] Children and Adults with Attention-Deficit/Hyperactivity Disorder (CHADD), "General Prevalence of ADHD," CHADD.org, accessed July 10, 2025, https://chadd.org/about-adhd/general-prevalence/.

in adulthood as people learn to address their symptoms through a variety of approaches.[5] The prevalence of ADHD is higher in boys than girls, with this disparity lessening somewhat in adulthood. In most cases, ADHD is considered a multifactorial disorder, where multiple biological and environmental risk factors cumulatively increase the likelihood of developing the disorder.

ADHD is genetic—estimated 77 to 88 percent heritability—and is considered a discrete diagnostic category. A reduction in neurotransmitters such as dopamine may play a key role in ADHD. Also, analysis of brain imaging data shows that individuals with ADHD have less activity in areas of the brain having to do with executive functions, such as the ability to control emotions, manage tasks, and make plans.[6]

Dr. Edward (Ned) Hallowell, one of the first doctors to write about ADHD and who was diagnosed with ADHD after completing his psychiatric residency at Harvard University, famously compared having an ADHD brain to a Ferrari engine with bicycle brakes. He discusses that attention is not just deficient but is actually variable. Hallowell suggests that it is actually "Variable Attention Stimulus Trait," or VAST.[7]

---

[5] Oliver Grimm, et al., "Genetics of ADHD: What Should the Clinician Know?" *Current Psychiatry Report*, 22(4) (2020): 18, https://doi.org/10.1007/s11920-020-1141-x.

[6] Kenneth Blum, et al., "Attention-deficit-hyperactivity disorder and reward deficiency syndrome," *Neuropsychiatric Disease and Treatment*, 4(5) (2008): 893–918, https://doi.org/10.2147/NDT.S2627.

[7] Edward Hallowell and John Ratey, "ADHD Needs a Better Name. We Have One." *ADDitude Magazine* (2025), https://www.additudemag.com/attention-deficit-disorder-vast/?srsltid=AfmBOoosxym8Ki5HOrEMn2V-NOMHVJ92OJSvLFhqhIb2d52aQgWstSK_7.

Many would suggest ADHD is not truly a disorder, but a variation of how brains function. In my opinion, the degree of disability experienced by those with basic function challenges warrants both classification as a disorder and the administration of psychiatric medication to relieve symptoms. Hallowell's description of a variable ability to attend seems more accurate and affirming of people with ADHD brains.

The key takeaway is that people with ADHD can hyperfocus and be extremely productive *if they are interested in the subject matter*, but if the task is not interesting, it can be nearly impossible to complete the job. Once engaged, they can't switch gears, especially if the second task is less intriguing. As a result of the varied ways ADHD may manifest its symptoms and impacts, it is often missed by family and professionals.

> **attention deficit disorder (ADD)**
> A term referring to individuals with the inability to attend (usage dropped in 1987).

Furthermore, there is confusion about the distinction between ADD and ADHD. The disorder is classified into three types: predominantly inattentive, predominantly hyperactive-impulsive, and combined. In my years of practice, I have never seen the predominantly hyperactive-impulsive presentation. Everyone has inattention and some people have external hyperactivity, but everyone has internal hyperactivity and impulsivity. Providers do not recognize that the inattentive person who does not display external hyperactivity is *mentally* hyperactive, experiencing multiple thoughts a minute. In the past, doctors considered this person to have attention deficit disorder (ADD). The American Psychiatric Association stopped using the term ADD in 1987, replacing it with ADHD.

The latest *Diagnostic and Statistical Manual of Mental Disorders* (DSM-5)[8] refers to ADHD as still having the three presentations listed above. I find it more helpful to use Dr. Daniel Amen's six types.[9] An interesting interpretation by Douglas Cowan, PsyD, LMFT, from the ADHD Information Library uses characters from the *Winnie the Pooh* children's stories to make Dr. Amen's types easier to understand and spot.[10] In the list below, I've replaced Amen's "Ring of Fire" (type 6) with a more common type that I've observed: "Owl."

1. **Tigger:** Inattentive, hyperactive, and impulsive; classic ADHD

   This type can't sit still, has trouble focusing, loses things, is distractible, is careless, is forgetful, has difficulty organizing activities, fails to follow through, avoids activities that are boring or hard, is restless, has difficulty waiting their turn, interrupts, and talks too much. This is classic ADHD and the character we associate with those four letters: "Bouncing is what Tiggers do best."

2. **Winnie the Pooh:** Inattentive, internal, and impulsive

   This type is disorganized, has low energy and motivation (unless it's about their interest—honey), and appears internally preoccupied. People with this presentation may be diagnosed later in life (more common in girls).

---

[8] American Psychiatric Association, ed., *Diagnostic and Statistical Manual of Mental Disorders, Fifth Edition, Text Revision (DSM-5-TR)* (American Psychiatric Publishing Inc., 2022).

[9] Daniel Amen, *Healing ADD: the Breakthrough Program that Allows You to See and Heal the 6 Types of ADD*, Berkley Publishing Group (2001).

[10] Douglas Cowan, "Different Types of ADHD: Inattentive ADHD in Scottsdale, AZ," ADHD Information Library (2017), https://adhd.newideas.net/.

They are often labeled lazy, unmotivated, and not smart. They may appear spacey, bored, and out of touch with reality. They are often late. On the inside, like Pooh, they are deep and kind.

3. **Piglet:** Inattentive, hyperactive, and anxious

   These people are often anxious or over-focused, have trouble shifting attention, are frequently stuck in loops of negative thoughts, are obsessive, worry excessively, are inflexible and sometimes argumentative, have difficulty shifting attention, hold grudges, and have a need for sameness. Piglet, however, bravely defends his friends and is creative, passionate, and loyal.

4. **Eeyore:** Inattentive, internally impulsive, and a ruminator; limbic ADHD

   Eeyore types present as depressed and inattentive. They exhibit chronic low-grade melancholy, are often negative, present low energy, communicate feelings of hopelessness and worthlessness, have low self-esteem, are often irritable, and engage in periods of social isolation. They may exhibit poor appetite and disrupted sleep patterns. When focused on their friends, Eeyore is authentic, caring, and can be a good listener.

5. **Rabbit:** Inattentive, over-focused, impulsive, and irritable

   Rabbits are seen as irritable and over-focused, inattentive, or aggressive. They think dark thoughts, present with mood instability, and are very impulsive. They may break rules, fight, be defiant, be rigid, have trouble shifting attention, and be disobedient. Poor handwriting and trouble learning is common. They often have a short fuse and difficulty distinguishing helpful corrections from insults. However, Rabbits are also sociable and ready to hop into action whenever their friends are in need.

6. **Owl:** Inattentive, internally impulsive, big picture person

Owls are highly intellectual and imaginative, not very focused on details, and make many spelling mistakes. An owl's purpose is to learn about the world around them, while figuring out what they want to do with their life. They are constantly learning new things and often see things in different ways than other people. Owls also become easily overwhelmed and need to retreat to their tree for rest. People presenting as Owl are also very creative and are excellent storytellers.

Most people display a combination of at least two of these subtypes. They might be hyperactive and outgoing while in public, but retreat to a more anxious, depressed, or irritable state in private. They may be the person who sees what others don't notice. What's important is that most people do not present as Tigger. Consider whether your mind is hyperactive or impulsive and you have trouble attending to boring but important tasks. Unfortunately, those who are more introverted, intelligent, and sometimes anxious or depressed often go undiagnosed by their family and practitioners. It is not uncommon for individuals to do very well in school until they must juggle multiple deadlines at once or need to complete too many boring or repetitive responsibilities.

People with ADHD are universally drawn to the "shiny object." They like to focus on what is interesting, novel, urgent, or scary. They are not inclined to address unstimulating duties, and this can lead to serious delays and, ultimately, an imbalance in their ability to be productive and take care of the necessary details of daily life. It was this long-term frustration that led Matt, in my introductory story, to feel suicidal. He knew what he was capable of, in theory; he just couldn't make himself apply his talent in a consistent manner that would ultimately produce an outcome that he was proud of. His self-esteem was understandably dangerously low.

Naturally, people who live with ADHD may also have additional mental health issues. Depression, anxiety, and other conditions show up in approximately 30 to 40 percent of those with ADHD. My experience is that when a person's ADHD is properly treated, their depression and anxiety often decrease or even cease altogether, as Matt experienced.

Imagine a child who is told multiple times a day that they've done something wrong: forgot their lunchbox, are late, didn't hand in the assignment (that was in their backpack), and more. After thousands of these incidents, the child becomes anxious. After tens of thousands of incidents, the child feels depressed that they are not able to perform at the level of their peers. This is often the moment when a health-care provider may be asked to prescribe antidepressants.

The power of proper treatment is profound, as evidenced by these quotes from two clients.

> *"It won't be an understatement to say everything is different. Finding acceptance and understanding helped me learn to love my brain and myself as I couldn't before 'the diagnosis.' The moment I stepped foot into the journey of addressing my ADHD (VAST) brain felt like putting on glasses for the first time and realizing the world wasn't blurry—my eyes were just made to see through a different lens."*

"Right now, even after taking medicine, everything has a different perspective: The hyperfocus is a superpower—I can absorb the subject of my attention and be attentive to the complexities, textures, intricacies, while at the same time envisioning the possibilities. The 'daydreaming' that still happens spontaneously at 37 years of age is the same as 'visualizing' positive outcomes and gaining the confidence to take certain actions. The distractibility or 'getting lost' on my way to accomplishing my missions is a process that allows me to venture outside of the straight line from 'point A to point B' and EVERYTIME I notice or learn something curious along the way."

ADHD DIAGNOSIS: ADULT SELF REPORT SCALE (ASRS) VS. FULL NEUROPSYCHOLOGICAL REPORT

Taking that first step to get diagnosed can be daunting. No one wants to be labeled or considered broken. On the other hand, if there isn't an actual diagnosis, a person may be prone to wonder if these issues are "all my fault" or "maybe I am just lazy, stupid, or crazy." There may be a fear of losing oneself or being forced to take medication. Very often, people with ADHD feel like they are treated like children who need extra reminders and accommodation to do basic tasks. However, they can also turn on their turbo focus and accomplish far more than the average person can in a concentrated period.

Generally, a great deal of struggle, shame, and failure have occurred before someone seeks diagnosis. Unfortunately, the professional world is not yet fully educated as to what ADHD is and how to treat it. It is not uncommon for a medical or mental health professional without sufficient expertise to do harm by providing misinformation, admonishing their client to just try harder, prescribing antidepressants, or worse.

"My family practice doctor told me he couldn't diagnose me, and I'd have to get a two-day, very expensive evaluation before we knew I had ADHD. He gave me Prozac and said because I had a master's degree, I probably didn't have ADHD."

Many believe that to be diagnosed with ADHD, a person must have a neuropsychological evaluation administered by a specially trained psychologist. In the United States, these evaluations can take four to eight hours and cost as much as $6,000. Naturally, this is prohibitive and reduces access to diagnosis. Worse, unlike the United Kingdom, Canada, and Australia, the United States does not have a set of national clinical practice guidelines for the treatment of ADHD. Many medical schools, nurse practitioner programs, and physician assistant educational programs do not offer courses on ADHD, and textbooks on ADHD have only recently been published. As a result, ADHD remains poorly understood and provider perspectives vary greatly. Practitioners feel underprepared and leery of prescribing stimulant medications. Most practitioners rely on the lists of criteria in the DSM-5-TR for diagnosing ADHD. Here is a summary[11]:

Diagnosis in Children and Teenagers

Diagnosing ADHD in children depends on a strict set of criteria: six or more symptoms of inattentiveness, or six or more symptoms of hyperactivity and impulsiveness.

---

[11] American Psychiatric Association, *Diagnostic and Statistical Manual of Mental Disorders*, Section II: Neurodevelopmental Disorders, 68–70.

Inattentiveness (Difficulty Concentrating and Focusing)

Main signs:

- ☀ having a short attention span and being easily distracted;
- ☀ making careless mistakes—for example, in schoolwork;
- ☀ appearing forgetful or losing things;
- ☀ being unable to stick to tasks that are tedious or time-consuming;
- ☀ appearing to be unable to listen to or carry out instructions;
- ☀ constantly changing activity or task; and
- ☀ having difficulty organizing tasks.

Hyperactivity and Impulsiveness

Main signs:

- ☀ being unable to sit still, especially in calm or quiet surroundings;
- ☀ constantly fidgeting;
- ☀ being unable to concentrate on tasks;
- ☀ excessive physical movement;
- ☀ excessive talking;
- ☀ being unable to wait their turn;
- ☀ acting without thinking;
- ☀ interrupting conversations; and
- ☀ little or no sense of danger.

To be diagnosed with ADHD, your child must also have:

☀ been displaying symptoms continuously for at least six months;

☀ started to show symptoms before the age of 12;

☀ been showing symptoms in at least two different settings—for example, at home and at school—to rule out the possibility that the behavior is not just a reaction to certain teachers or to parental control;

☀ symptoms that make their lives considerably more difficult on a social or academic level; and

☀ have symptoms that are not just part of a developmental disorder or difficult phase and are not better accounted for by another condition.

Diagnosis in Adults

Diagnosing ADHD in adults is more difficult because there's some disagreement about whether the list of symptoms used to diagnose children and teenagers also applies to adults.

In some cases, an adult may be diagnosed with ADHD if they have five or more symptoms of inattentiveness, or five or more symptoms of hyperactivity and impulsiveness listed in diagnostic criteria for children with ADHD. As part of the assessment, the specialist will ask about present symptoms. However, under current diagnostic guidelines, a diagnosis of ADHD in adults cannot be confirmed unless symptoms have been present from childhood. If a person finds it difficult to remember whether they had problems as a child, the specialist may wish to see old school records, or talk to parents, teachers, or anyone else who knew the client well as a child.

For an adult to be diagnosed with ADHD, their symptoms should also have a moderate effect on different areas of their life, such as:

☀ underachieving at work or in education;

☀ driving dangerously;

☀ having difficulty making or keeping friends; or

☀ having difficulty in relationships with partners.

If a person's problems are recent and did not occur regularly in the past, they're not considered to have ADHD. This is because it's currently thought that ADHD cannot develop for the first time in adults.

There are several versions of assessment tools that subjectively measure symptoms of inattentiveness, hyperactivity, and impulsiveness. The Connor and Vanderbilt Scales are the most administered assessment tools for children. My preference is to use the Adult Self-Report Scale, v1.1 (2005), designed by the World Health Organization (WHO), see Figure 1.[12] In 2020, the WHO updated the self-assessment tool and now offers a simpler and yet very accurate version of this extremely useful tool, ASRS-5, that offers 91.4 percent accuracy for the diagnosis of ADHD in adults and is used in Canada and Australia, see Figure 2.[13]

---

[12] Attention Deficit Disorder Association, "Adult ADHD Questionnaire: Self-Report Scale (ASRS-V1.1)," add.org, accessed July 14, 2025, https://add.org/wp-content/uploads/2015/03/adhd-questionnaire-ASRS111.pdf.

[13] ADHD Quiz Australia, "Adult ADHD Self-Report Screening Scale (ASRS)," ADHDQuizAustralia.com.au, accessed July 14, 2025, https://adhdquiz.com.au/asrs/.

ADULT ADHD SELF-REPORT SCALE (ASRS-V1.1) SYMPTOM CHECKLIST

Patient: _____ Date Completed: _____

Please answer the questions below, rating yourself on each of the criteria shown using the scale on the right side of the page. As you answer each question, place an X in the box that best describes how you have felt and conducted yourself over the past 6 months. Please give this completed checklist to your healthcare professional to discuss during your appointment.	Never	Rarely	Sometimes	Often	Very often
PART A					
How often do you have trouble wrapping up the final details of a project, once the challenging parts have been done?	☐	☐	☐	☐	☐
How often do you have difficulty getting things in order when you have to do a task that requires organization?	☐	☐	☐	☐	☐
How often do you have problems remembering appointments or obligations?	☐	☐	☐	☐	☐
When you have a task that requires a lot of thought, how often do you avoid or delay getting started?	☐	☐	☐	☐	☐
How often do you fidget or squirm with your hands or feet when you have to sit down for a long time?	☐	☐	☐	☐	☐
How often do you feel overly active and compelled to do things, like you were driven by a motor?	☐	☐	☐	☐	☐
PART B					
How often do you make careless mistakes when you have to work on a boring or difficult project?	☐	☐	☐	☐	☐
How often do you have difficulty keeping your attention when you are doing boring or repetitive work?	☐	☐	☐	☐	☐
How often do you have difficulty concentrating on what people say to you, even when they are speaking to you directly?	☐	☐	☐	☐	☐
How often do you misplace or have difficulty finding things at home or at work?	☐	☐	☐	☐	☐
How often are you distracted by activity or noise around you?	☐	☐	☐	☐	☐
How often do you leave your seat in meetings or in other situations in which you are expected to stay seated?	☐	☐	☐	☐	☐
How often do you feel restless or fidgety?	☐	☐	☐	☐	☐
How often do you have difficulty unwinding and relaxing when you have time to yourself?	☐	☐	☐	☐	☐
How often do you find yourself talking too much when you are in social situations?	☐	☐	☐	☐	☐
When you're in a conversation, how often do you find yourself finishing the sentences of the people you are talking to, before they can finish it themselves?	☐	☐	☐	☐	☐
How often do you have difficulty waiting your turn in situations when turn taking is required?	☐	☐	☐	☐	☐
How often do you interrupt others when they are busy?	☐	☐	☐	☐	☐

Figure 1. Adult ADHD Self-Report Scale v1.1.

ASRS-5: Adult ADHD Self-Report Scale

Instructions

This self-assessment is designed to help identify symptoms of ADHD in adults.

Please answer the questions below, rating yourself on each of the criteria shown. As you answer each question, select the box that best describes how you have felt and conducted yourself over the past 6 months.

		Never	Rarely	Sometimes	Often	Very Often
1	How often do you have difficulty concentrating on what people say to you, even when they are speaking to you directly?	0	1	2	3	4
2	How often do you leave your seat in meetings or other situations in which you are expected to remain seated?	0	1	2	3	4
3	How often do you have difficulty unwinding and relaxing when you have time to yourself?	0	1	2	3	4
4	When you're in a conversation, how often do you find yourself finishing the sentences of the people you are talking to before they can finish them themselves?	0	1	2	3	4
5	How often do you put things off until the last minute?	0	1	2	3	4
6	How often do you depend on others to keep your life in order and attend to details?	0	1	2	3	4

Scoring

The maximum possible score is 25

Total Score: [   ]

- A score of **14 or higher** suggests the possible existence of ADHD.
- A cutoff score of 14 correctly identifies **91.4%** of adults with ADHD and **96% without.**

Source: https://pmc.ncbi.nlm.nih.gov/articles/PMC5470397/

While these scores suggest the possibility of ADHD, it's important to note that this is not a definitive diagnosis. Only a qualified healthcare professional can diagnose ADHD after a comprehensive evaluation.

adhdquiz.com.au   Page 1 of 1

Figure 2. Adult ADHD Self-Report Scale 5.

THE VALUE OF SCREENING FOR ADULTS WITH ADHD

Research suggests that the symptoms of ADHD can persist into adulthood, having a significant impact on the relationships, careers, and even the personal safety of people who may suffer from it. Because this disorder is often misunderstood, many people who have it do not receive appropriate treatment and, as a result, go through life operating below their full potential. Thus, it is helpful to destigmatize, better assess, and emphasize the benefits of treatment for those with ADHD in the adult population.

Statistics

Statistically, the negatives are very concerning, and the positives are not to be missed. (See Chapter 3.) Some facts:

- ☀ Eleven percent of all children in the US have ADHD.
- ☀ ADHD is observable in four-year-olds, although the initial onset is usually around seven to eight years.
- ☀ It is twice as common in boys as in girls.[14]
- ☀ Females often present as inattentive and are the most overlooked group when it comes to diagnosis and proper treatment.

---

[14] U.S. Centers for Disease Control and Prevention, "Data and Statistics on ADHD," CDC.gov (2024), https://www.cdc.gov/adhd/data/index.html.

☀ Teens with ADHD receive four times as many traffic citations and have 36 percent more car accidents than their peers without ADHD.[15]

☀ Teens with ADHD who have an auto accident are seven times more likely to have a second accident.

☀ Although the national high school drop-out rate is 15 percent, 21 percent of teens with ADHD skip school and 32 to 38 percent drop out before finishing high school.[16]

☀ Untreated, ADHD life expectancy is reduced by 11 to 13 years.[17]

☀ The rate of persistence of ADHD into adulthood varies across studies. A review of seven North American controlled prospective follow-up studies found high rates of symptomatic persistence (60 to 86 percent).[18]

---

[15] Allison E. Curry, et al., "Motor Vehicle Crash Risk Among Adolescents and Young Adults With Attention-Deficit/Hyperactivity Disorder," *Journal of the American Medical Association Pediatrics*, 171(8) (2017): 756–763, https://doi.org/10.1001/jamapediatrics.2017.0910.

[16] Children and Adults with Attention-Deficit/Hyperactivity Disorder, "ADHD and Long-Term Outcomes," CHADD.org, accessed July 15, 2025, https://chadd.org/about-adhd/long-term-outcomes/.

[17] Russell Barkley, PhD, "How ADHD Affects Life Expectancy," *ADDitude Magazine*, March 25, 2025, https://www.additudemag.com/adhd-life-expectancy-video/?srsltid=AfmBOorD4pyMxP-qgc437LRqzFLl1c-8goXdYR3AULRoBLlsFxG4LWwNm.

[18] Mariya V. Cherkasova, et al., "Review: Adult Outcome as Seen Through Controlled Prospective Follow-up Studies of Children With Attention-Deficit/Hyperactivity Disorder Followed Into Adulthood," *Journal of the* American *Academy of Child and Adolescent Psychiatry*, 61(3) (2022): 378–391, https://doi.org/10.1016/j.jaac.2021.05.019.

ADHD may be easier to identify in women during adulthood, where they may become aware of their symptoms and self-refer for assessment.[19] A worsening of ADHD symptoms and impairments may be more noticeable during adult transition periods, such as moving away from the family or beginning university/employment.

Some adults with ADHD may experience "hyperfocus" and engage in specific activities for many hours, when the activities are highly interesting. Mind wandering and mental restlessness may also be present. Adults can present with more subtle hyperactivity, such as feeling restless and not being able to relax. Impulsivity in adults may result in excessive spending, binge eating, interpersonal conflict, risk-taking, addictions, talking excessively, or interrupting others.

And, of course, these behaviors may be related to something else entirely. Adults with ADHD are equally likely to meet criteria for one or more co-occurring disorders and experience significant impairments in daily life, such as difficulties in romantic relationships or emotional control.

A recent review suggested three reasons for the perceived onset of ADHD in adulthood:

1. Symptoms not previously considered significant due to lower environmental demands, the presence of support in the environment, or factors such as high IQ;

---

[19] Susan Young, et al., "Females with ADHD: An expert consensus statement taking a lifespan approach providing guidance for the identification and treatment of attention-deficit/hyperactivity disorder in girls and women," *BMC Psychiatry*, 20 (2020): 404, https://doi.org/10.1186/s12888-020-02707-9.

2. Failure to identify ADHD in the presence of other conditions; and

3. Symptoms present in childhood but not previously identified or attended to.[20]

"There is nothing 'wrong' with you. Our brains just work differently from others and given the right tools, a strong support system, therapy and guidance, along with medications if deemed necessary by a therapist or prescriber, it is possible to function in a way that might be very different from the way you've been functioning. You can feel successful and competent. Let go of the stigma attached to having to take medication. Let go of all the negative things you've been told about your ADHD. You wouldn't criticize someone with diabetes for taking insulin to control their blood sugar. It can save their life. Having ADHD and taking medication to help you control your impulsiveness is not much different. And maybe most importantly, understand that change is a process, and be patient with yourself. You'll get there."

CHAPTER 2 PEARLS

1. Many people will look anxious and/or depressed, but the underlying reason may be ADHD.

2. *Variable Attention Stimulus Trait* is a better descriptor for people who have an inconsistent ability to

---

[20] J. J. S. Kooij, "Updated European Consensus Statement on diagnosis and treatment of adult ADHD," *European Psychiatry*, 56 (2019): 14–34, https://doi.org/10.1016/j.eurpsy.2018.11.001.

concentrate, but we'll stick with ADHD for consistency's sake.

3. People with ADHD are not all physically hyperactive; everyone in *Winnie the Pooh*, except Christopher Robin and Kanga, has ADHD.

4. Physical hyperactivity is not a required characteristic of ADHD, but everyone has mental hyperactivity.

5. The ADHD ASRS-v1.1 (full) or ASRS-5 (shortened) assessment is a valuable initial screening tool.

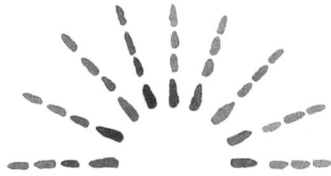

CHAPTER 3

The ADHD Personality— Heartfelt Creativity

Before treatment, I was a lot less confident in myself and my diagnosis.

After, I was able to fully understand my unique strengths and challenges and recognize that some of the challenges are a part of my disorder and not internalize them as "bad" parts of myself.

Before treatment, my emotions ran a big portion of my life.

After treatment, I have coping skills, and I can recognize the emotion without letting it overcome me and ruin my day, if not weeks.

Before treatment, I had a hard time recognizing why relationships felt like so much work and can be so challenging for me.

After treatment, I'm able to express who I am to people in my life, so they are better able to understand me and meet me where I am at, making relationships a bit more manageable to me.

Before treatment, when trying to initiate a hard conversation with my partner, I was more likely to say things off the cuff and in a heated way.

After treatment, I'm more able to slow down and think about what I want to say and how I'd like to say it, making conflict resolution easier.

It might seem odd to consider that there is a personality associated with ADHD. In reviewing my experience, my clients have demonstrated the positive attributes of people living with neurodivergence—so much so that I am literally delighted to start each and every day of work.

Let's start by considering famous people generally known or thought to have had ADHD. As you read this selective list compiled from several websites,[21] think of the positive associations you have with their success:

[21] Mia Barnes, "10 Famous People Who Had ADHD and Made It Their Superpower," Body + Mind blog, October 31, 2024, https://bodymind.com/famous-people-who-had-adhd/.

ADDitude Editors, "11 Neurodivergent Grammy Nominees," *ADDitude Magazine*, March 26, 2025, https://www.additudemag.com/slideshows/12-neurodivergent-grammy-nominees/?srsltid=AfmBOoohScWEanPW-6z1i1j34drZXf75_Vx_EotlR-quvE4LrU_entxCH.

"Famous People with ADHD/AS," ADHD-Support.org.uk, accessed August 4, 2025, https://adhd-support.org.uk/famous.htm.

"33 Celebrities Who've Opened Up About Having ADHD," WikiGrewal, accessed August 4, 2025, https://www.wikigrewal.com/famous-people-who-have-adhd/.

Inventors, Entrepreneurs, and Scientists: Henry Ford, Thomas Edison, Walt Disney, Leonardo da Vinci, Alexander Graham Bell, Orville and Wilber Wright, Sir Isaac Newton, Albert Einstein, Marie Curie, and Bill Gates

Actors: Robin Williams, Sylvester Stallone, Suzanne Somers, Will Smith, Dustin Hoffman, Whoopi Goldberg, Emma Watson, Tracey Gold, Bill Cosby, Cher, Jim Carrey, George Burns, Channing Tatum, Trevor Noah, Johnny Depp, Karina Smirnoff, Bex Taylor-Klaus, Paris Hilton, Zooey Deschanel, Ryan Gosling, Cara Delevingne, and Cameron Diaz

Musicians: Ludwig van Beethoven, Adam Levine, Brittany Spears, Justin Timberlake, Sam Fender, Solange Knowles, John Lennon, Wolfgang Amadeus Mozart, Elvis Presley, Billie Eilish, Ariana Grande, and Lady Gaga

Leaders: Abraham Lincoln, Robert F. Kennedy, John F. Kennedy, Benjamin Franklin, and Woodrow Wilson

Authors: Agatha Christie, George Bernard Shaw, Jessica McCabe, and Dev Pilkey

Athletes: Michael Phelps, Simone Biles, Babe Ruth, Mohammad Ali, and Michael Jordan

---

S. J. Tsai, "Top 17 Famous Scientists With ADHD That You May Not Know," Sci Journal, updated April 18, 2024, https://www.scijournal.org/articles/famous-scientists-with-adhd.

Priya Florence Shah, "21 Famous Neurodivergent People in History and Today," Blog Brandz.com (2024), https://www.blogbrandz.com/tips/famous-neurodivergent-people/#content.

Clara Muriel, "90 Famous People with ADHD: Struggles & Strengths," Very Special Tales.com (2023), https://veryspecialtales.com/famous-people-with-adhd/.

This list makes it clear that having ADHD does not prevent success or fame. Perhaps ADHD helped propel these famous people into their careers. They had to be extremely driven and able to hyperfocus on their unique skills and passions, whether inventing a vehicle or communication device, creating world-renowned music, producing great literature and theater, performing at the Olympic level, or leading a nation during a tumultuous time.

I have observed these valuable traits associated with my ADHD clients over the years:

- Forgiving
- Creative
- Sensitive
- Compassionate
- Empathic
- Warmhearted
- Charismatic
- Intuitive
- Trusting
- Passionate
- Charming
- Visionary
- Dreamer
- Visual learner
- Fast thinker
- Insightful
- Inventive
- Flexible
- Loyal
- Tenacious
- Risk-taker
- Multi-talented
- Humorous
- Spontaneous
- Fun-loving
- Energetic
- Enthusiastic
- Athletic
- Optimistic
- Resilient

It is obvious why I love working so much with these genuine people. I have found that people with ADHD tend not to bully or judge with the intent to harm or mock. They tend to be particularly empathic and able to feel the other person's pain. Wouldn't you want that capacity in your life or on your team?

The language we use to describe ADHD matters, and one of the most painful aspects of living with ADHD is being judged by others and internalizing that judgment. Reframing the discussion is a good place to start. See Table 1 for language suggestions.

INSTEAD OF:	USE:	INSTEAD OF:	USE:
Suffer	Lives with	**Manage a child**	Care for; support
Suffering	Struggles	**Manage behavior**	Guide
Label	Diagnosis	**Deficit**	Difference; neurodiverse
Behavior	Symptoms; traits; characteristics	**Treatable**	Thrive with treatment and support[22]

Table 1. Reframing the conversation.

The research on ADHD mood issues examines emotional dysregulation and rejection-sensitive dysphoria. So much focus is placed on negative traits—centering on inattention, forgetfulness, impulsivity, and hyperactivity—that as a person living with ADHD, it is easy to become overwhelmed with a negative self-opinion. You probably have received feedback

---

[22] ADHD Evidence Project, "Are There Positive Aspects to ADHD?" ADHDEvidence.org, April 4, 2022, https://www.adhdevidence.org/blog/are-there-positiveaspects-to-adhd-2.

> **emotional dysregulation**
> Difficulty controlling the intensity, duration, or expression of emotions, causing reactions that may be inappropriate or disproportionate to the situation.
>
> **rejection sensitive dysphoria (RSD)**
> Extreme emotional sensitivity to the perception of being rejected, criticized, or teased. *See Chapter 5.*

since childhood that includes messages such as "You don't care" because you . . . "are late," "didn't complete the task or assignment," "are interrupting," or "are fidgeting." People who hear things like this, and who have a hefty dose of rejection sensitivity, may find themselves being overly self-critical with little to no recognition of their many strengths and insights.

Hallowell reframes the three major components of ADHD. He suggests that the flip side of *distractibility* is "curiosity"; the opposite of *impulsivity* is "creativity"; and that of *hyperactivity* is "energy."[23]

Imagine if we could recognize that the person with ADHD who is described as an *inattentive, impulsive, hyperactive disruptor* is instead an *energetic, creative seeker of truth*?

Using this lens, I can assure you that you are awesome. You are kind, have a great sense of humor, pick up on cues the rest of us miss, can come up with new ideas to address problems that others find unsolvable, and demonstrate a striking ability to be resilient even in the face of repeated failure. Your ability to accept others for who they are and see the positive in hard situations is notable. As evidenced by the list of successful famous people with ADHD, there is no limit to your ability to achieve greatness.

---

[23] Edward (Ned) Hallowell, "Positives of ADHD," AccuTrain YouTube channel (2017), https://www.youtube.com/watch?v=JfAGo9VGEzo.

"For most of this journey, I struggled to get to a place of acceptance. Language is everything. The medical language currently used makes it feel like 'sickness'—I hope to see medical professionals and leaders become more thoughtful of the way language can be the root cause of much of the dysfunction and intentionally work toward adopting more positive or at least neutral language around any type of neurodiversity and not just ADHD. I can understand how we continue using certain language as it's what we've used for decades, but if the ultimate goal is meaningful progress and true healing, then there should be a change in course, that starts with the language."

CHAPTER 3 PEARLS

1. People with ADHD have dozens of positive attributes, including creativity, heartfulness, kindness, nonjudgmental attitude, and unique problem-solving ability.

2. Professionals and the public at large need to become better educated on how to use more positive descriptors when referring to people living with ADHD.

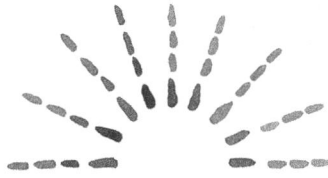

CHAPTER 4

ADHD: Four Letters, Five Characteristics: Inattention, Memory, Impulsivity, Hyperactivity, and Rejection Sensitivity

I can't tell you how relieved I am to be told just like the book says. "So you mean I'm not lazy, stupid or crazy?" It's been 10 years of trying different antidepressants for my supposed depression and anxiety and arguing with my doctors that something else was wrong. Even after I explained that everything takes me twice as long, they told me I'm clearly intelligent and not hyperactive, so I don't have ADHD and should use better time management. I'm constantly getting feedback that if I just try harder, I could produce more of the high-quality work that I hand in intermittently. I feel like a veil has lifted, although I still struggle to get started at

35

times. Once I do, I am finishing projects in less than half the time I needed for completion, before I took stimulants. I have more energy, am sleeping better, and my girlfriend tells me I am a lot more fun to be around. It has been amazing.

The common image of a young boy jumping up and down, not listening, skews our view of the many possible ways ADHD presents. As discussed in Chapter 2, ADHD shows up in a multitude of ways. Hyperactivity and impulsiveness are the most noticeable symptoms when a person has external hyperactivity. However, the most common characteristic is problems attending to important tasks. This disrupts the lives of most individuals with ADHD. Nearly everyone with ADHD has trouble getting started on boring work, not getting distracted, and completing the whole job. Less obvious are the issues with memory, impulsivity, and inner hyperactivity. Hyperactivity and impulsivity often retreat internally to the less noticeable mental overstimulation. People tend to develop strategies to remember key tasks. What is hardly understood at all is the emotional dysregulation that accompanies this condition.

In his excellent article on executive functions, Dr. Thomas E. Brown describes six clusters of aspects of the ADHD brain[24]:

Activation

Getting started is the most perplexing part of ADHD. Most people depend on last-minute urgency to overcome their procrastination. Sadly, it is the proverbial "stick"—a negative

---

[24] Thomas E. Brown, "The Brown Model of Executive Function Impairments in ADHD," BrownADHDClinic.com, accessed June 7, 2025, https://www.brownadhdclinic.com/brown-ef-model-adhd.

consequence—that gets them focused and going. Common household chores and multistep work or school projects suffer and may take weeks to complete.

Once you've finally begun, the next hurdle is the challenge of prioritizing tasks. Planning for the completion of the project means coming up with a road map or design and a supply list, considering costs, time requirements, and labor, before climbing to the top of the steep mountain. Once the ascent starts, it will often become apparent that the mountain is actually only a hill.

Focus

Staying focused on a task can be as challenging as starting, as people with ADHD find themselves easily distracted. The classic example of experiencing a sudden uncontrollable distraction is referred to as a "squirrel." People with ADHD juggle dozens of thoughts and feelings at a time. They struggle to block out distractions; background noises, internal or external, which are disruptive and take a great deal of effort to ignore. This is part of why so many people with ADHD suffer from exhaustion. It takes a tremendous amount of effort to concentrate on important, although boring, tasks.

Distraction causes significant problems in school, work, driving, daily activities, relationships, and self-care. The reverse can also be true; the person's ability to hyperfocus at the expense of other necessary tasks may leave important actions uncompleted. Hyperfocus often happens with electronic devices, phones, video games, and computers. Being an effective attender requires the ability to sort through external and internal stimuli and screen out the unimportant and distracting.

We all experience this to some degree or another, but with ADHD, this is pervasive and the root of much frustration and, unfortunately, failure.

Effort

Many people with ADHD have significant problems with day-time drowsiness and are unable to stay alert without regular physical or mental engagement. Sitting for long periods of time can make it nearly impossible to pay attention to the topic at hand. Daytime fatigue usually begins with poor sleep patterns, a common affliction of living with ADHD. Falling asleep can be difficult, and often those with ADHD wake during the night and are unable to fall back asleep. When they do fall asleep, they may sleep so deeply that they struggle to wake up and have difficulty transitioning into their daytime schedule. This is why a short-acting stimulant can be extremely helpful early in the day.

People with ADHD tend to have slower processing speeds, so completing tasks may take longer. Reading and writing can be particularly slow, so academic accommodation for ADHD may include extra time to finish exams and assignments. Finally, shifting from one task to another can be very difficult. Parents of children with ADHD have learned to give multiple signals of upcoming change to help them transition more smoothly. Often adults with ADHD have learned to set several alarms to help them transition from sleeping to waking or from one task to another.

Emotion

The most surprising and poorly understood aspect of ADHD is mood dysregulation. Brown's description of symptoms related to managing frustration and modulating emotions points to the core of this problem. He describes people who have ADHD as having a low threshold for irritability.[25] Dr. William Dodson calls this constellation of symptoms "rejection sensitivity dysphoria (RSD),"[26] described as a rush of emotions that replace all other feelings, as though the brain becomes flooded with a perception that the individual has done wrong (see Chapter 5).

Despite the exceptional ability to empathize and recognize another's upset feelings, there is little tolerance for the negative self-interpretation that others do not concur with. This feeling can be very intense and can take over the ability to self-regulate. This can lead the person with ADHD to speak abruptly or impulsively and not consider another person's feelings or thoughts. Sometimes people with ADHD are described as overly sensitive and unable to regulate feelings of discouragement or sadness. Some describe it as though their mind has been invaded like a computer virus. It impacts every part of their thoughts and emotions.

Memory

ADHD includes problems with working memory, such as recalling directions and general difficulty with planning, organizing, and carrying out daily chores.

> **working memory**
> The amount of information that can be kept in mind and used in the execution of future cognitive tasks.

---

[25] Brown, "The Brown Model of Executive Functions."

[26] William Dodson, "New Insights into Rejection Sensitive Dysphoria," *ADDitude Magazine* (updated 2025), https://www.additudemag.com/rejection-sensitive-dysphoria-adhd-emotional-dysregulation/?srsltid=AfmBOor2eqHcyjKz5zZNufc9-uLNgwXEeTmy62A1ofnqgW4zPYXvaueT.

To engage in these types of tasks successfully, one must hold onto some facts while working on others, ultimately needing to integrate the first set of facts into the task. Brown compares this to a computer's RAM combined with its file manager and search engine. People with ADHD have challenges retrieving information needed to respond to the presenting situation.[27]

You must be able to hold onto the communications shared with you and respond to them before jumping in with your own opinions or experiences. An inability to do this can cause issues in relationships when the partner without ADHD feels that their experience is not attended to due to the excessive need for the person with ADHD to express their feelings first.

Reading requires active working memory use, since the text builds on itself and relies on the reader retaining information from previous sentences and paragraphs. Math also requires the ability to hold a sequence of operations. Those with ADHD are thus often challenged to perform well in these subjects at school or in life.

Action

Most behaviors have a beginning and end—a decision to act and another to inhibit. To make successful and safe decisions, we must act and stop acting depending on both danger and importance. Take crossing a street: It is clear when it's a good time to act and when to stop, properly balancing urgency and safety.

Social interactions can be more challenging for people living with ADHD, who have difficulty monitoring meaning and

---

[27] Brown, "The Brown Model of Executive Functions."

self-regulating their behaviors. In social situations, they may interrupt, be distracted and not respond at all, or delay answering direct questions.

Also, the ability to quickly assess another person's expectations or actions can be skewed. People with ADHD may pick up on another's emotional distress before a neurotypical person does, while also making misjudgments about how to have a sensitive conversation that involves confrontation or disappointment. They might miss important details or over-focus on less important ones. There can be misperceptions as to how others feel or react, and a decreased ability to tune into their own emotions or recognize how they are coming across.

The opposite can also occur. People with ADHD and anxiety may be excessively focused on how others react, leading to heightened shyness and an inability to engage in social situations. People with ADHD often do not enjoy being the center of attention. They may be excellent performers on stage but dread having to talk with the audience afterward.

In summary, the five components of ADHD—inattention (including activation, focus, and effort); memory; impulsivity; hyperactivity; and mood (or rejection sensitive dysphoria)—make this a complex, multifaceted condition. It is also why professionals often misdiagnose people as having anxiety and depression, missing the underlying ADHD when there is no overt hyperactivity or impulsivity and emotional dysregulation is the primary presenting symptom.

"When I listened to Dr. Dodson describe rejection sensitive dysphoria, I cried. I couldn't believe this wasn't just my super-critical, oversensitive brain. Just knowing that it's a part

of ADHD was such a huge relief. I felt a lot kinder toward myself and realize that my big heart needs to find more space for myself and not just always focus on everyone else."

CHAPTER 4 PEARLS

1. Procrastination—trouble getting started—is the most common ADHD symptom.

2. Hyperactivity and impulsivity may be present internally only and not be recognizable by others.

3. Emotional dysregulation, or rejection sensitive dysphoria, is the second most common debilitating aspect of ADHD.

4. ADHD is commonly misdiagnosed as anxiety or depression.

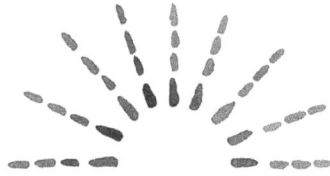

CHAPTER 5

Rejection Sensitive Dysphoria: Criticism, Emotional Regulation, Over-Functioning, Perfectionism, and Self-Esteem Issues

I was relieved, sad, angry, but mostly relieved. It explained a lot about the heartache. Learning about rejection sensitive dysphoria made sense of a lot of behaviors I could not make sense of before. Since I was young, I always felt like everyone was going to leave me if I didn't behave a certain way, or if I was too "difficult" or too much. This feeling could be para-lyzing to me at times, and I never knew where it came from. I'd rack my brain to figure out what trauma had caused this in my life. When I found out it was mostly due to RSD, I felt relieved. I now had something to work with and a label for this pattern of thinking. This knowledge has given me the ability to change the thought patterns so I'm now more confident and don't really struggle with those once paralyzing fears anymore.

Mood dysregulation is not a symptom that we associate with ADHD, but in recent years, Dodson's writings on RSD have gone viral, exposing many more people to the term. His update on RSD in *ADDitude Magazine* describes this poorly understood aspect of ADHD. I've summarized the article here, and I encourage you to carefully read the full article in its entirety, as RSD is the second most disabling aspect of ADHD.[28]

Rejection sensitive dysphoria is "unbearable" emotional pain caused by rejection or criticism (perceived or real) that is not relieved with therapy. While not a formal diagnosis, RSD is a very common expression of emotional dysregulation, a brain-based symptom of unbearable pain, often seen (and misunderstood) in adults. The individual's response to RSD is often disproportionate to the triggering event, which could be external (criticism, including constructive, or rejection, including teasing or perceived disrespect) or internal (self-criticism or negative self-talk).

This pain can feel physical, like the person has been punched. It can start in the teen years and lead to suicidal thinking and mood disorders. Conversely, it can also be expressed outwardly, presenting as rage toward anything or anyone that appears to be at the root of the pain. This may wax and wane many times a day.

---

[28] Dodson, "New Insights Into Rejection Sensitive Dysphoria."

Signs of RSD vary: negative, self-deprecating comments; problems maintaining relationships; and ruminating thoughts and actions. Unlike depression, these incidents come and go, but the emotional responses can be very extreme.

RSD is not recognized as a symptom of ADHD in the US, but emotional dysregulation is used to diagnose ADHD in Europe. We don't yet have formal research on treatment options; however, Dodson has obtained positive results (about 60 percent) using guanfacine and clonidine—approved ADHD treatments—for RSD. In his words, "This observation strongly indicates that RSD is neurological and not due to a lack of skills. Skills do not come in pill form."[29]

The article then provides details about diagnostic criteria, history, and treatment options, as well as the limited published research and the cool reception the research has received from many clinicians.

Not surprisingly, when I asked my clients to comment on what has changed in their lives since being treated for ADHD, they mentioned RSD more than any other characteristic. Even though it's frustrating to have trouble attending due to procrastination and distraction, feeling criticized by either another or oneself appears to be the most painful aspect of living with ADHD.

"I had the best conversation with my 11-year-old daughter about RSD today. She was having big, tender feelings after her friends told her they didn't want to audition for a play she hadn't written yet (but it was VERY real in her head).

---

[29] Brown, "New Insights into Rejection Sensitive Dysphoria."

They said they were going along with it earlier because they didn't want to hurt her feelings but now, they wanted to do something else. She was telling me she knew it was overreacting, but she felt super hurt and upset and was sure they didn't want to do it because they thought all sorts of negative things about her. I introduced her to RSD and told her it's the evil goblin whispers that seep into our thoughts sometimes and try to convince us that everyone is in a huge secret club behind our backs, and they are sitting around talking shit about us. And something about a 'magic brain' (her term for brains with ADHD) wants to stick to those thoughts and make them echo louder and louder until you get so upset you can't move, or you decide to go blow up a relationship or quit a project or a club or a job. I told her it wasn't just her, and I had those too. I told her sometimes I need help to step way back and look at all the evidence I have that it is not actually true. And often, expressing that I am getting turned around by the echoes of shitty thoughts in my own head to the people I trust and know are worthy of my vulnerability makes it way easier to blow the echoes away and get back to being myself in my life. She looked at me with huge eyes and said, 'You have that, too? I thought it was just me.'"

"I used to be stuck in the wind tunnel often and for days at a time, immobilized by the guilt and shame I felt. I never had a name for how I felt when RSD hits me; I thought I must have been crazy or maybe everyone felt this way. It was a relief to know what it is and how to manage it. I know for myself it won't completely go away, but I have the tools to get myself out of that wind tunnel faster, and I feel stronger for it."

"It made a huge impact on me, as far as recognizing that there is an actual name for the cluster of symptoms that

have been lifelong for me, with no reasonable explanation (I have no history of severe trauma, had positive parenting, etc.). These symptoms included wanting to please others, performance anxiety with the smallest of things, and hyper-sensitivity to (unverified) interactions/behaviors in others that might indicate dislike, judgment, or rejection of me. So, knowing this is essentially a neuro/biological thing in my brain generally made me see it differently."

"Learning about RSD had a very positive impact. I felt alone and anxious thinking that I was always overreacting and too sensitive. Knowing that it is a normal symptom of ADHD helps me manage and understand why I react to certain situations, and I have worked hard to learn more about how to self-sooth and communicate to my partner when I am feeling especially sensitive. We've learned together that I usually just need a good hug, or affirmation that it is okay that I'm feeling overwhelmed and upset. Usually, it is the worst for me after a long day of RSD, and it is a 'final straw' that has really pushed me over the edge to where I feel like I cannot handle my emotions."

In *How to ADHD*, Jessica McCabe offers excellent ideas for understanding and responding to "Emotional Dysregulation, the impaired ability to control one's emotional response, which can lead to extreme and/or disproportionate reactions that are not necessarily appropriate to the situation."[30] She offers some suggestions about this least understood (and often most destructive) aspect of ADHD.

---

[30] Jessica McCabe, *How to ADHD: An Insider's Guide to Working with Your Brain (Not Against It)* (Penguin Random House, 2024).

When overwhelmed with emotions, people with ADHD often describe feeling flooded or taken over, like with a computer virus. They experience wave after wave of feeling that can't be stopped. People observing someone having such a big reaction may respond with advice: "Just stop crying," "it's nothing," "don't be scared," "calm down," or "you're being so dramatic." People who regularly experience, and express, these big feelings often learn to hide them to avoid unraveling into a panic attack because of the enormity of what they are feeling.

ADHD brains don't regulate emotions well; they hit harder and last longer, and people with ADHD tend to be more reactive to emotions than others. This reactivity impacts how someone with ADHD responds to the world, and how the world, in turn, reacts to the person. They must adopt a variety of coping mechanisms. When someone suggests they know what the person with ADHD is feeling ("Aren't you worried?" "I'll bet you're happy about that."), people with ADHD may learn to simply agree.

Because RSD is not recognized as a key component of ADHD, people are instead diagnosed with anxiety and/or depression and are given antidepressants rather than treatment for ADHD. Most health professionals do not understand this form of emotional dysregulation and are not prepared to address it.

It may help to better understand how the core attributes of ADHD contribute to mood dysregulation. Many people with ADHD experience increased emotional impulsivity, with difficulty pausing and inhibiting their first reaction when emotions begin to flair. Once in a reactive (or flooded) state of mind, it is difficult to refocus one's attention.

Also, when feeling emotionally "hot," it can be difficult to access executive functions requiring the ability to calmly think through multiple steps. In general, cognitive abilities decline as emotions rise, so people with ADHD may not remember what should happen next or may impulsively choose the wrong step. McCabe says that people with ADHD skip past "yellow," going straight from "green" to "red" when responding to rising emotions.

Unfortunately, this behavior can result in being labeled as too sensitive, immature, or selfish. People are told that their meltdowns are shameful and wrong. When moving from one mistake, obstacle, or deadline to another, there is no time to return to a more regulated emotional baseline. These are times when people with ADHD may say or do things they later regret, resulting in reprimands at school or work or serious problems with family members who don't understand their expressions of sadness, fear, rejection, or even desire beyond what is expected for the situation.

The opposite can also be true: People with ADHD may be told they are too joyful, excited, or humorous; they seem too big and too loud; and their decision-making skills may appear flawed. The risk of being criticized for overreacting often results in the suppression of emotions. This can lead to the masking of feelings and, sometimes, self-medicating with alcohol, drugs, and/or food.

On a more positive note, people with ADHD may learn to control their environment and themselves to be less likely to overreact. This can be as simple as choosing where to socialize or sit in class, reframing situations into a positive spin, or using breathing techniques and mindfulness strategies.

Dealing with mood dysregulation may require several steps, the first being to just notice and not judge our emotions.

1. Label Your Emotions

Sometimes it's hard to distinguish between a thought and a feeling. "I think you hate me" is a thought and a judgment. "I'm afraid our friendship is over" is a feeling. Deciding how "hot" something is—green, yellow, or red—might be a clue as to whether to let it go (green), address it before it gets worse (yellow), or wait until you calm down to talk about it (red).

I really appreciate the work of Marshall Rosenberg on nonviolent communication.[31] He emphasizes the importance of offering empathy to *yourself* first and then figuring out the core feeling—often it's loss, sadness, hurt, or fear. Then try to sort out what unmet need is associated with the feeling. In the example above, the unmet need might be for connection or understanding. Finally, make a doable request of yourself or the other individual. For our example: "Would you be willing to get together tomorrow for an hour and talk about our friendship? I'd like to feel more connected."

2. Make Space for Your Emotions

Many people living with ADHD have been told their emotions are wrong, so making space for them is vital for learning to validate your feelings. Wait to act, to be clear about what you feel and to allow time to process what happened. It's helpful to ask for time to think and feel. You may want to explore your feelings; drawing, writing, or talking with another person can help you express yourself.

---

[31] Marshall B. Rosenberg, *Nonviolent Communication: The language of life*; (PuddleDancer Press, 2015).

3. Use Your Emotions

Feelings are indicators that we might need more or less of something. Sometimes our strong emotions can help us push past fears, motivate others, or be effective problem-solvers. Sometimes the gut gets a clear message before the brain does. Paying attention to emotions can help navigate situations more effectively. Feeling things strongly makes us feel alive and should not be avoided. It's wonderful to be fully present; this contributes to overall happiness, even when experiencing something difficult.

A profound tip from McCabe: **Expressing *thoughts* might result in problems, but expressing *feelings* will generally help with connecting.** And from Rosenberg: Communication is most effective and powerful when it's built on genuine emotion. "People connect better with what you say if you make them *laugh* or if you make them *feel*."[32]

4. Find Your Emotional Balance

Opening the doors to big feelings can let in an absolute flood, which is uncomfortable, decreases our options for responding, and may result in actions we regret. We can be proactive by controlling our thoughts, behavior, and environment to adjust the "emotional volume."

Some ways of dealing with the constant barrage of input and settling your emotional distress:

- Practice meditation.
- Have a plan for emotionally difficult situations.

---

[32] Rosenburg, *Nonviolent Communication*.

- Talk with a friend.

- Step away.

- Direct your attention to something you can control (my favorite: helping someone else).

Feelings are signals. It's important to allow those signals to come through and know how to interpret what they mean. Sometimes our emotions will swallow us regardless of our coping skills because life is hard and ADHD makes it harder. Grief happens and so does trauma. Try to remind yourself that they are time-limited and ask for support.

RSD can be treated with medications that are roughly 60 percent effective. Guanfacine and Clonidine have been successfully used to decrease the intensity of negative self-talk and help with sleep. I refer to the medications as a "brain balm." Generally, they are taken before bed; an extended-release version seems to work best. Some providers actually prefer to start with these medications and follow with a stimulant. They tend to calm the brain's excessive inner chatter down, which can help to improve attention. They are, however, not a substitute for stimulant medications.

"I am reminded of how much of my life is impacted by this 'condition.' It describes many of my reactions to things and is the main thing I want to address and work on. Understanding that it is organic in nature and often associated with ADHD brain structure is reassuring. Knowing why I react the way I do to certain things is quite comforting."

"It emphasizes to me the idea of myself and others with ADHD, tuning into multiple things at once—when there is

one thing (TV volume) that is too much, it can feel overstimulating. This seemingly small impairment can seem a lot more significant in the moment, before properly processing."

"Learning about RSD helped me gain a lot of self-confidence and encouraged me to start saying 'no' more often."

"In my line of work, we encourage everyone to be 'friendly with errors'; however, I wasn't able to embrace my own errors in the same way I did for others. Learning about RSD helped me to be friendly with my own errors and use them as a learning experience for myself and others. Sharing the mistakes I made, pointing them out to someone who may do something similar, makes me feel better and stops me from continuously repeating the scenario in my head."

"Knowing about RSD also makes me more open to feedback, specifically criticism, because I know the negative things I'm thinking and feeling are self-inflicted. When I feel rejected or embarrassed because of something someone said, I try to replay the scenario and parse out what I added or assumed that made me feel the way I do. I try to figure out if the message I received was actually the message they intended to deliver."

"I am also very uncomfortable in large groups/new places and am always worried about embarrassing myself. I used to use alcohol as a crutch to help me feel more comfortable in these situations, which never actually made me feel calmer or at ease. Now, when I'm invited to a social event with more than four to five people, I consider how I really feel about going—am I excited, anxious, looking forward to it, only saying yes because my husband wants to go? I talk to my husband about how I feel and decide if it's something

I want or need to attend. I'm more likely to say, 'no thanks' when I want to, and he's better able to help me feel comfortable when I do attend larger gatherings."

CHAPTER 5 PEARLS

1. RSD is the perception that you have failed or are being criticized.

2. In Europe, emotional dysregulation is considered a core component of ADHD.

3. Decrease a reactive response by first focusing on what you are feeling, making space for the feeling, and pausing before responding.

4. Tell the other person how you are feeling and ask for what you need.

5. Guanfacine and Clonidine can help decrease the intensity of RSD symptoms.

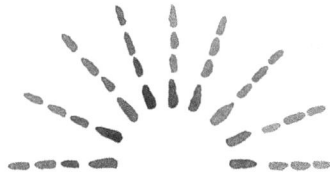

CHAPTER 6

Genetics—Guidance from Your Genes

Having the ability to do genetic testing made me trust the process so much more! Not only did I get to know my body and my brain more, but there was proof of more than just the ADHD medication that did or did not work for me.

Getting the genetics data changed my entire treatment plan. I discovered I had been taking an anti-depressant for years that wasn't working at all because my body is a super-fast metabolizer, and my depression wasn't getting better. That was incredibly disappointing but also a relief to be able to know that there were other options, and I was able to find a drug that works for me.

It was the most eye-opening thing for me! It was proof to myself that this was REAL; I was not making things up in my head, that I was actually struggling, and some things were truly harder for me. I feel like I know myself better than I ever have, and I can take control and have power over what's going on inside me.

GENETIC TESTING

ADHD is a genetic condition that responds well to treatment with stimulant medications 85 to 90 percent of the time. Additionally, it is helpful to uncover what other genetic and biochemical root causes may be contributing to an individual's difficulties with focus and mood regulation. There are several genetic markers that can help us better understand the underlying reasons a person may struggle with their ADHD symptoms.

pharmacogenetic
The study of how genetic differences among individuals cause varied responses to a drug.

Identifying certain pharmacogenetic markers can shed light on whether specific drugs will be effective and if there is a higher risk of adverse events from those drugs. Providers can tailor treatment plans to each patient based on test results, including genetic variations that predict changes in how brain functions will react. Understanding how quickly a person metabolizes medications helps avoid issues such as ineffectiveness, drug-resistance, and drug interactions. This process is a more objective, evidence-based guide to help providers select the right medications for their patients.

Genetic testing is not just for people struggling with a non-responsive medication regimen. It can help speed up the choice of the correct medication and dosage for new clients. It may also reduce or eliminate the roller coaster ride of medication resistance or prevent a plateau in symptom relief down the road. Current genetic testing addresses a variety of disorders, including depression, anxiety, and bipolar disorder. Indicators for addressing ADHD, OCD, PTSD, and schizophrenia are also being developed.

Here are some of the specific genes we can test for today and their impact on mental health:

MTHFR

Methylenetetrahydrofolate reductase (MTHFR) is an enzyme responsible for converting folic acid to L-methylfolate needed for serotonin, norepinephrine, and dopamine synthesis (neurotransmitters critical for concentration and self-regulating action and mood). They also create immune cells, process hormones like estrogen, produce energy, and detoxify chemicals.

Those with defective MTHFR genes (estimated 20 to 70 percent) have an impaired ability to produce the MTHFR enzyme. This can make it more difficult to break down and eliminate synthetic folic acid and substances like heavy metals.

Since folic acid can't be converted into the usable form, it can build up in the body, raising levels of homocysteine, an amino acid associated with a higher risk of cardiovascular disease. This also affects the conversion to glutathione, a potent antioxidant needed to remove waste.

Individuals with low MTHFR enzyme activity may present with elevated homocysteine levels, associated with depression, inflammation, dementia, autism, heart disease, birth defects, difficult pregnancies, miscarriage, neural tube defects, cleft palates, Down's syndrome, and, potentially, an impaired ability to detoxify.

We are still learning, but there is strong evidence that it can increase risks of cancer, cardiovascular disease, and fetal development problems and may also contribute to or exacerbate problems like autoimmune disease and mental issues.

Since people with ADHD have a decreased level of active dopamine and norepinephrine, and a MTHFR deficiency creates a deficit in L-methylfolate, it is critical to test everyone with ADHD to determine if they have this genetic deficiency. If they do, then supplement with high quality methylated folate.

Depression and Anxiety

There is growing evidence of a role for various folate forms in the prevention and treatment of depression. In fact, there is compelling evidence that treatment with an L-methylfolate agent would not only avoid the potential risks of antidepressants in pregnancy but would also confer important benefits to pregnancy and child outcomes as well, such as prevention of major birth defects and longer-term neurodevelopmental outcomes. L-methylfolate may be an effective form of folate supplementation to target depression and may be more readily absorbed in the brain than other forms.[33]

> **monotherapy**
> The use of a single drug to treat a condition.

Fava and colleagues demonstrated that L-methylfolate is significantly superior to placebo for the treatment of major depressive disorder in patients who didn't

---

[33] Alan L. Miller, "The methylation, neurotransmitter, and antioxidant connections between folate and depression," *Alternative Medicine Review*, 13(3) (2008): 216–226, https://pubmed.ncbi.nlm.nih.gov/18950248/.

respond to antidepressant therapy alone. Several other studies of L-methylfolate monotherapy in depressed populations have found that patients experienced significant improvement in depressive symptoms with no drug-related adverse events. Initial studies indicate that L-methylfolate may be safe and effective for treatment of depression, especially in those vulnerable to medication-related adverse events and those who are folate-deficient.[34] While most over-the-counter methylfolate products are compounded with calcium, methylfolate is best absorbed when compounded with magnesium. To my knowledge, the only product that currently meets this criterion is known as EnLyte® by JAYMAC Pharmaceuticals. A typical starting dose is about 6 milligrams. Consult your provider before using methylfolate.

COMT

Catechol-O-Methyltransferase (COMT) is an enzyme responsible for the breakdown of dopamine in the frontal cortex of the brain. One gene variant, Val/Val, will increase COMT enzyme activity, decreasing frontal cortex dopamine and working memory. Dopaminergic stimulants may lead to improvements in executive function for Val/Val allele carriers compared to Met/Met allele carriers, who may need to use stimulants cautiously. Val/Met carriers are the dominant variant and will have the average rate of dopamine breakdown.

> **allele**
> An alternative form of a gene that may occur at a particular place on a chromosome.

---

[34] Maurizio Fava, Richard C. Shelton, and John M. Zajecka, "Evidence for the use of 1-methylfolate combined with antidepressants in MDD," *Journal of Clinical Psychiatry*, 72(8) (2011): e25, https://pubmed.ncbi.nlm.nih.gov/21899813/.

Many people present with a MTHFR deficiency plus increased activity in the COMT gene, resulting in faster disintegration of existing dopamine. These ADHD clients will generally require a much higher dose of stimulant to compensate for their lower levels of dopamine. This partially explains why the range of proper dosing is so varied. I have clients who take from 2.5 milligrams to over 90 milligrams per day. Knowing about your COMT gene will help determine an effective dose of stimulant medication. It will explain why a standard starting dose of 10 milligrams of Ritalin or Adderall may not be the best way to begin.

Spoiler alert: This will be covered in Chapter 8, but always start low, at 5 milligrams, and go up slowly by 2.5-milligram increments to determine the ideal dose. This will avoid overmedication from the start.

ADRA2A

> **adrenergic**
> Activated by or involving adrenaline or an adrenaline-like substance.
>
> **cytosine (C) and guanine (G)**
> Two of the four recognized DNA bases. The others are adenine (A) and thymine (T).

ADRA2A encodes the α-2A adrenergic receptor, a norepinephrine receptor. This is thought to mediate the effects of norepinephrine in the prefrontal cortex of the brain and regulate symptoms of ADHD. Research has shown that the C/G gene variant will show an improved response to Ritalin for inattentive symptoms of ADHD in children and adolescents, compared to those with the C/C genotype. It does not appear to have any influence on Adderall.

This means if a person has the C/G variant, they are more likely to respond to Ritalin than if they have the C/C type. If a person newly diagnosed with ADHD presents with ADRA2A C/C, the provider might want to consider starting treatment with Adderall first.

CYP P450 Enzymes: CYP2D6, CYP2C19, CYP2B6, CYP1A2, CYP2C9

Cytochrome P450 enzymes are involved in the pharmacokinetic metabolism of many clinically used psychiatric drugs. There is a graduated range of medication metabolism rates, starting with the slowest or poorest metabolizer, up to the fastest, an ultra-rapid metabolizer.

> **pharmacokinetics**
> The characteristic interactions of a drug and the body.

CYP2D6 is responsible for the metabolism and elimination of approximately 25 percent of clinically used drugs. A deficiency of this enzyme is inherited as an autosomal recessive trait; about 7 percent of Whites and

> **autosomal recessive trait**
> A genetic trait requiring that both parents contribute an abnormal gene.

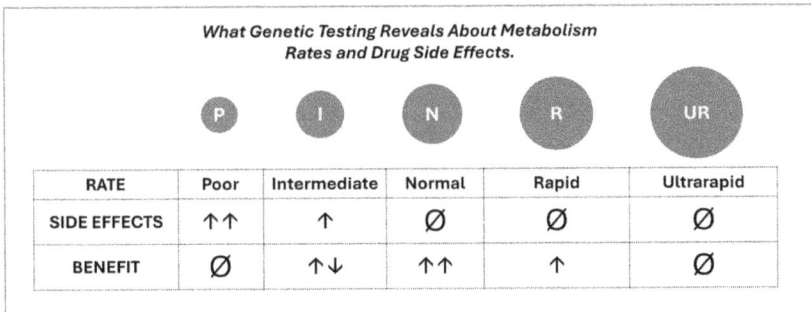

What Genetic Testing Reveals About Metabolism Rates and Drug Side Effects.				
P	I	N	R	UR
RATE Poor	Intermediate	Normal	Rapid	Ultrarapid
SIDE EFFECTS ↑↑	↑	Ø	Ø	Ø
BENEFIT Ø	↑↓	↑↑	↑	Ø

Figure 3. Genetic Testing, Metabolism Rates, and Drug Side Effects.

1 percent of Asians are classified as poor metabolizers. Those who are poor or intermediate metabolizers are likely to experience side effects and few or no benefits when using a medication that is largely metabolized through this genetic pathway. On the other hand, a person who is a rapid or ultrarapid metabolizer is likely to have little to no benefit but few side effects (see Figure 3). A commonly prescribed antidepressant, fluoxetine (Prozac), uses this pathway. This explains why one only has a 25 to 33 percent chance of efficacy without side effects when first starting Prozac and other selective serotonin reuptake inhibitors (SSRIs).[35]

Since many people take antidepressants before, during, and after starting stimulant medications, it is extremely helpful to know how their genetic makeup impacts their treatment and use of medications. It is not uncommon to discover that the side effects someone experiences are due to being a poor or intermediate metabolizer for the prescribed medication. Conversely, one might learn that due to rapid metabolization, the medication is mostly or entirely ineffective. Many providers have been taught to only conduct genetic testing after multiple drug failures. If the client is already on medication, it will confirm their experience or explain their side effects. If they are not yet on medication, it narrows the field of which drug is likely to be most effective and can eliminate many months of trial and error. I have seen clients who have been on the wrong medication for years prior to doing genetic testing. For individuals with MTHFR deficiency, supplementing with L-methylfolate can be life changing.

---

[35] Megan Kane, "CYP2D6 Overview: Allele and Phenotype Frequencies," *Medical Genetics Summaries*, Victoria M. Pratt, Stuart A. Scott, Munir Pirmohamed, et al, (ed. 2021; rev. 2025), https://www.ncbi.nlm.nih.gov/books/NBK574601/.

WHY IS GENETIC TESTING
NOT THE STANDARD OF PRACTICE?

The traditional trial-and-error treatment and increased incidence of preventable health complications due to adverse drug events is very unfortunate. Genetic data helps reduce guesswork, identify side

> **psychotropic**
> Medications that act on the mind.

effects, and make personalized treatment decisions possible. Unfortunately, genetic testing for psychotropic medications is not yet the standard of care. One supposition is that this is, in some way, controlled by "big pharma," as it is in their best interest not to have precise testing modalities. Sadly, this encourages extensive trials of the wrong drug.

Generally, clinicians are taught that this testing is still experimental, and it is not recommended until the client has endured several drug failures. This makes no sense when considering the enormous benefit in choosing the right drug early in a person's treatment. Panels of tests are offered for a few hundred dollars, and it is possible to order individual MTHFR blood or saliva tests through your healthcare provider. There are also some companies that will send you an at-home kit. Since 75 percent of my clients have a MTHFR variance, it is highly likely that you may be dealing with some version of this genetic deficiency that contributes directly to ADHD and mood disorders.

"The genetic testing gave me some confidence about which group of meds would be more likely to be helpful for ADHD, depression, and anxiety. I guess if I'd seen a different provider, they might have started me on an antidepressant that caused side effects."

"Knowing that there are certain drugs I tolerate well/ unwell was interesting (especially in retrospect) to how I could manage both my ADHD and other things."

"Learning about my genetic data was incredibly interesting! It was reassuring to have an explanation for those medications I'd previously tried and why they didn't work for me. I also learned that exercise can be as beneficial for me as medication, which led to a huge 'aha' moment in realizing I'd self-medicated with exercise for years and my mental health took a big downturn when I was no longer training as a collegiate athlete."

CHAPTER 6 PEARLS

1. Genetic testing should be the standard of care for anyone being considered for psychotropic medication.

2. Methylenetetrahydrofolate reductase (MTHFR) deficiency occurs in over 60 percent of the population and contributes to medical and physical health problems.

3. Supplementing with L-methylfolate can significantly improve one's mood and ability to concentrate.

4. Knowing in advance whether you are a slow, normal, or fast metabolizer allows you and your provider to make good medication choices.

5. Only 25 to 30 percent of people who try an antidepressant will be an ideal genetic match; 65 to 70 percent of people will experience no benefit or have a side effect that interferes with the efficacy of the medication.

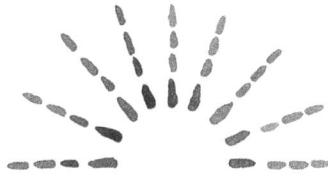

CHAPTER 7

Functional Medicine: Discovering Sources of Imbalance in Your Brain and Body

At the time I went to see Maggie, I had been to five different practitioners. I'd tried medications, supplements, counseling, sleep devices, and exercise. Nothing really made much improvement in my ability to concentrate and my chronic low mood. We did lab work, and she was so excited that I had so many imbalances. This seemed strange, but after three months of addressing my vitamin D, iron, and zinc deficiencies, I felt significantly better. I started sleeping more, my energy improved, I could pay attention and complete tasks better, and my mood was happier. No one else had asked what my vitamin D and iron levels were, never mind my zinc count. She explained that these micronutrients help to make neurotransmitters. I knew it helped with bone growth, but I didn't realize it also helps to build muscles and skin and is important for my mental health. My mood went from lousy to pretty well most days. It was amazing. Once I had more energy, I started exercising and making better food choices. I could pay attention for much longer.

TREATING ADHD WITHOUT MEDICATIONS

According to the Institute for Functional Medicine (IFM), functional medicine is a systems-based approach to identify and then address the root causes of disease, recognizing that a person's illness may be made up of many symptoms or differential diagnoses.[36] For example, a functional medicine-trained practitioner might look at a depressed person and consider numerous biological factors in addition to the usual social and psychological stressors, such as early childhood adverse events, racial or other marginalized injustice, trauma, and current challenging life circumstances.

According to IFM, "Functional medicine treats the whole person, addressing the unique physical, mental, and emotional needs of each patient. Clinicians bring together the entire complement of modern scientific tools, including a deep understanding of biology, physiology, genetics, social and environmental determinants of health, and the vital connection between mental and physical well-being. It is this combination of focusing on individual patients and applying a multi-faceted treatment path that delivers transformational results."[37]

---

[36] The Institute for Functional Medicine, "Functional Medicine," IMF.org, accessed June 5, 2025, https://www.ifm.org/. Used with permission.

[37] Institute for Functional Medicine, "Functional Medicine Restores Healthy Function by Treating the Root Causes of Disease," IFM.org, accessed

When I started as a psychiatric nurse practitioner in 2013, I was skeptical about the value of psychotropic medications, antidepressants, stimulants, and more. I hoped that we could address most mental health issues with diet, therapy, and exercise. After observing the enormous significance that stimulants and, sometimes, antidepressant medications have made in many of my clients' lives, I took a deeper look at how well they worked and how to determine the best stimulant, dose, and frequency for each client. The results were truly profound, and for many people, stimulants will offer lifelong support. At the same time, I longed to reach deeper into the root causes of mental health problems.

In 2017, at the Integrative Medicine for Mental Health conference, I met Dr. James Greenblatt, the founder of Psychiatry Redefined and author of numerous books on functional medicine. Greenblatt opened my eyes to the fascinating world of uncovering the underlying reasons for anxiety, depression, and, sometimes, concentration issues and hyperactivity. I began asking all my clients to do lab testing in addition to the genetic testing they were already doing, resulting in interesting discoveries. Often, getting a person's vitamin D, zinc, iron, or cholesterol levels up to an optimal level was all that was needed to greatly improve their mood or help them sleep better. These changes occurred slowly over weeks and months, but when maintained, clients frequently saw permanent relief from their symptoms.

Greenblatt impressed upon me to "test and not guess." First, consider what biochemical, genetic, and environmental causes are contributing to the individual's problem. Using a drug to

June 19, 2025, https://www.ifm.org/functional-medicine. Used with permission.

increase a person's neurotransmitters is an inadequate response to a multifaceted problem. If a person suffers from MTHFR/ L-methylfolate deficiency, supplements are a good strategy to boost their mood and ability to concentrate. If a person is anemic, provide guidance that includes eating more iron-rich foods. If a person's vitamin D is low, inform them of the value of taking good-quality vitamin D3 with vitamin K2, which aids the absorption of vitamin D.

I also learned that there are other contributors, like gut and environmental health. It just makes sense to explore and treat as many root causes as possible. If the standard approaches of diet, therapy, exercise, and select supplements and medications don't work, then look more deeply. Could mold, Lyme, glyphosate, heavy metals, yeast, or gut issues be exacerbating the disruptive symptoms? Obviously, we can't test for everything, but a comprehensive initial panel will help eliminate many of the most common imbalances. It's also very motivating to have a measurable value that can be addressed by diet or supplementation rather than some vague notion that vitamins might be helpful. When a 13-year-old client of mine had all 35 lab values come back in the optimal range, I asked her mother what she fed her child. Her response:

> "Well, we don't eat any processed food, there's a small portion of protein in every meal, and we love our berries. In fact, I make berry pie several times a week. We have berry pie for breakfast, snacks, and dessert. Finally, I grew up in the south and I make sure we have cooked greens with every dinner. My daughter loves a whole bag of spinach sauteed in garlic and lemon juice. She has a soup bowl full of greens nearly every day."

Imagine if we all ate like this lucky child! This client's diet included protein, antioxidants, iron, vitamins, minerals, and fiber and was also low in processed foods and the range of additives that those include. She still needed a small dose of Ritalin to help with her attention issues, but her overall constitution was excellent.

ENVIRONMENTAL RISK FACTORS

Several environmental factors that may contribute to the risk of developing ADHD have emerged. Comprehensively reviewed in the World Federation of ADHD International Consensus Statement,[38] these include exposure to toxicants such as lead, phthalate, organophosphate pesticides, long-term maternal use of Tylenol during pregnancy, and prenatal exposure to the antiepileptic drug Valproate. Among the findings: While prenatal exposure to maternal smoking has been linked to an increased incidence of ADHD, this effect is significantly reduced when adjusting for a family history of ADHD, suggesting a link to an underlying genetic predisposition rather than a purely environmental risk. Research on prenatal and birth complication events as potential risk factors for ADHD found that preterm babies under 32 weeks of age and those with a birth weight of under 3.3 pounds are at risk for developing ADHD. Maternal obesity, hypertension, preeclampsia, and hypothyroidism during pregnancy have also been associated with increased risk of ADHD. A number of large-scale studies have linked the risk for ADHD to nutrient deficiencies. These include lower overall blood levels

---

[38] Stephen V. Faraone, et al., "The World Federation of ADHD International Consensus Statement: 208 Evidence-based conclusions about the disorder," *Neuroscience and Biobehavioral Review*, 128 (2021): 789–818, https://doi.org/10.1016/j.neubiorev.2021.01.022.

of ferritin and omega-3 polyunsaturated fatty acids in individuals with ADHD, compared with non-ADHD controls, and the association of lower maternal vitamin D levels with increased risk of ADHD in offspring.

There are also a range of situational/environmental factors that can substantially increase the risk for development of ADHD. These factors include intrauterine exposure to maternal stress (e.g., death of a close relative during pregnancy), trauma (e.g., sexual abuse), physical neglect (particularly for ADHD inattentive type), and psychosocial adversity (e.g., lowered family income, out-of-home care, paternal criminality, or maternal mental disorder).

THE ROLE OF LIFESTYLE CHANGES, THERAPY, AND COACHING IN ADDRESSING ADHD

Since there is so much concern about taking stimulants, it is important to review research on ways to treat ADHD without medications. Regardless of whether medications are provided, it is equally important to seek the root causes of biological and genetic imbalances that contribute to ADHD symptoms. The Australian ADHD Professionals Association (AADPA) published an excellent summary of the current research on non-pharmacological interventions for ADHD.[39]

Behavioral interventions include:

Lifestyle changes: Although little research has been done on the potential benefits of lifestyle changes for people

[39] Australian ADHD Guideline Development Group, *Australian Evidence-Based Clinical Guideline For Attention Deficit Hyperactivity Disorder (ADHD), First Edition*, 2022: 100–124, https://aadpa.com.au/guideline/.

with ADHD, AADPA encourages health-care providers to advise clients about the importance of a balanced diet, good nutrition, regular exercise, and quality sleep for all clients.

Cognitive Behavior Training: Research used in AADPA's analysis of cognitive behavior training (CBT) shows only limited positive impact for hyperactivity symptoms. Inattention and social skills were not shown to benefit from CBT.

Parent/Family Training: Parent/family training should be offered to families of children with ADHD with low to moderate certainty.

Neurofeedback (electroencephalography (EEG)): The benefits of neurofeedback for parent- or teacher-reported ADHD were inconsistent in children and adolescents. Benefits were shown for inattention symptoms based on parent report but not teacher or clinician report; and no benefits for parent or teacher were reported. For ADHD hyperactivity/impulsivity symptoms in adults, the evidence was inconclusive.

ADHD Coaching: The review of the research showed the potential that ADHD coaching may help support executive functioning, ADHD symptoms, self-esteem, well-being, and quality of life. Additionally, respondents reported being satisfied with their coaching and being able to maintain their gains. However, there was substantial variation across the studies, including coach training, program delivery (group or individual), duration, and outcomes assessed. Further research is required to determine its overall effectiveness.

In summary, the use of behavioral interventions does not appear to have a significant impact on treating ADHD.

Providing therapeutic counseling and coaching with medication and nutritional treatments may offer more benefits.

NUTRITIONAL AND ENVIRONMENTAL WELLNESS

There are many root causes of depression that a functional medicine practitioner can help you detect, treat, and heal: nutrient deficiencies, hormonal imbalances, food allergies and sensitivities, and environmental toxins. Biological components could include imbalances in vitamin D, B12, iron, zinc, or fatty acid; hypothyroidism; prediabetes; or a history of heavy antibiotic use. Often, perimenopausal and menopausal women discover that an estrogen deficiency leads to significant mood swings. Premenstrual irritability is well known; addressing this with nutrients can also combat what may be 25 percent of a woman's state of mind each month. Food allergies can contribute to difficulties with concentration, mood, and sleep, and environmental toxins can severely impact one's mental health, such as mold, glyphosate, lead, and air pollution.

> **pediatric autoimmune neuropsychiatric disorders associated with streptococcus (PANDAS)** Early childhood exposure to strep, followed by issues with mental health.

In addition to biological, hormonal, and environmental root causes, infections can weaken our immune systems and our ability to combat mental and physical health conditions: Lyme disease, toxoplasmosis, COVID-19, E. coli, and pediatric autoimmune neuropsychiatric disorders associated with streptococcus (PANDAS). Whether bacterial, viral, or fungal in origin, these conditions often prove difficult to address and require very specialized treatment.

The so-called "Gut-Brain Axis" has been well established. Most of our neurotransmitters are made in the gastrointestinal tract. Increasing evidence has associated gut microbiota with both gastrointestinal and extra-gastrointestinal diseases. Dysbiosis and inflammation of the gut have been linked to several mental illnesses, including anxiety and depression. Probiotics can restore normal microbial balance and therefore have a potential role in the treatment and prevention of anxiety and depression. Treating gluten or dairy sensitivity may also offer much needed relief from chronic mental health issues.

> **dysbiosis**
> An imbalance in the gut's microbiota—the microscopic organisms of your digestive tract.

In the age of COVID-19, we are more aware of the impact of loneliness, trauma, and social determinants of health. Access to healthy food, air and water quality, education, neighborhood safety, socioeconomic status, education, race, and gender all contribute to one's mental health considerations. These, too, would be considered when looking at mental health through a functional medicine lens. Finally, the basics, such as sleep, exercise, and diet, contribute enormously to a person's mental health.

When addressing ADHD from a functional medicine perspective, it is vital to consider the context of the person's life. Where are they living, do they have support, what are they eating, how much sleep and exercise do they get? Furthermore, what do their genetics and labs reveal that can be addressed right up front? Are they dealing with toxins that need to be cleared?

When treating ADHD, stimulant medications can be life-changing, since they will boost two critical neurotransmitters—norepinephrine and dopamine—quickly, but a person wishing to build a solid foundation for their future and possibly no longer need methylphenidate or amphetamines should find a practitioner experienced in or open to functional medicine root causes. Greenblatt recommends testing for anyone seeking to improve their mental health, see Table 2.

INITIAL RECOMMENDED LABORATORY TESTS

TEST TYPE	USED TO IDENTIFY
Functional medicine blood panel	Complete metabolic profile, complete blood count (CBC), lipids, hemoglobin A1c, high sensitivity C-reactive protein, ferritin, iron, vitamin D, vitamin B12, copper, magnesium, ceruloplasmin, zinc, and thyroid stimulating hormone, T3, free T3, and T4.
Genetic testing (blood or saliva test): As discussed in Chapter 5, especially looking at MTHFR.	People who may be slow or fast dopamine metabolizers and those who are not candidates for selective serotonin reuptake inhibitors, along with several other common psychotropic medications; it can also comment on the efficacy of methylphenidate (Ritalin) as a stimulant choice.
Organic acid testing (OAT) (urine test): This detects imbalances, toxicity, and inflammation and can indicate the functional need for specific nutrients, diet modification, antioxidant protection, and detoxification.	Comprehensive metabolic snapshot of patient's overall health with 75 markers; provides an accurate evaluation of intestinal yeast and bacteria. Abnormally high levels of these microorganisms can cause or worsen behavior disorders, hyperactivity, movement disorders, fatigue, and immune function. Includes markers for vitamin and mineral levels, oxidative stress, neurotransmitter levels, and markers for oxalates, which are highly correlated with many chronic illnesses. Strongly recommended as an initial screening in addition to the blood and urine testing recommended in this chart.

Table 2. Recommended Test Types.

TEST TYPE	USED TO IDENTIFY
Kryptopyrrole test (urine test): Aids in detection of pyrrole disorder, characterized by a dramatic deficiency of zinc, vitamin B6, and Omega-6.	**Pyrrole Disorder** Also known as pyroluria, kryptopyrrole, Mauve disorder, or kryptopyroluria. Poorly understood and relatively unknown condition that can make ADHD and most mental health issues much worse. Biochemical imbalance involving an abnormality in the synthesis and metabolism of hemoglobin. May be purely genetic or acquired through environmental and emotional stress; very common in people with leaky gut syndrome and those who have required repeated antibiotic use.
Hair mineral/ heavy metal testing	Accumulations of heavy metals in the body, disrupting the balance of essential nutrients, and becoming toxic to organ systems. Certain elements (calcium, chloride, cobalt, copper, fluoride, iodine, iron, lithium, magnesium, manganese, phosphorus, potassium, selenium, sodium, sulfur, and zinc) are vital for proper body function. Heavy metals such as aluminum, arsenic, cadmium, mercury, and lead are toxic and interfere with the body's ability to function.

Table 2. (*continued*).

Just like plants need key nutrients, such as nitrogen, phosphorus, and potassium, we depend on the availability and balance of core nutrients. Testing, not guessing, which micronutrients are out of balance can help to create a pathway to healing.

There is very little research comparing a strictly functional medicine approach, devoid of any stimulant medication, and treating ADHD with stimulants only. Anecdotally, I can confirm that the greatest positive change I've observed is in deploying a combination of four treatments: stimulants, micronutrients (including diet and supplements), supportive strategies, and therapy, particularly those therapies that are trauma-informed and teach mindfulness. Most often, newly diagnosed individuals will benefit from starting on stimulants right away, and then are better able to commit to, and benefit from, addressing their nutritional imbalances by using their improved focus and energy. Once nutritional imbalances have gained purchase, building better habits, employing time management strategies, and working therapeutically on underlying trauma and emotional issues enables the person to establish new routines and have a better understanding of their deeper strengths and abilities. It is awe-inspiring to help these individuals recognize their core value as creative, intelligent, resilient people who can be successful, generous, and kind.

MAKING SENSE OF TREATMENT PRIORITIES

The ADHD Evidence Project uses facts "to improve the lives of people with ADHD by curating, disseminating, and promoting scientifically researched and evidence-based conclusions about the disorder to patients, families, and clinicians."[40] Founded by Stephen Faraone, PhD; the organization offers a list of ADHD treatments based on the quality of the evidence that determines their efficacy.

The take-away message is that stimulant medication has the biggest effect, and other approaches offer some benefit and should be explored. It is, however, vital that the person be given the opportunity to trial medications and should not be afraid

[40] The ADHD Evidence Project, "Get to know ADHD," accessed June 5, 2025, https://www.adhdevidence.org/.

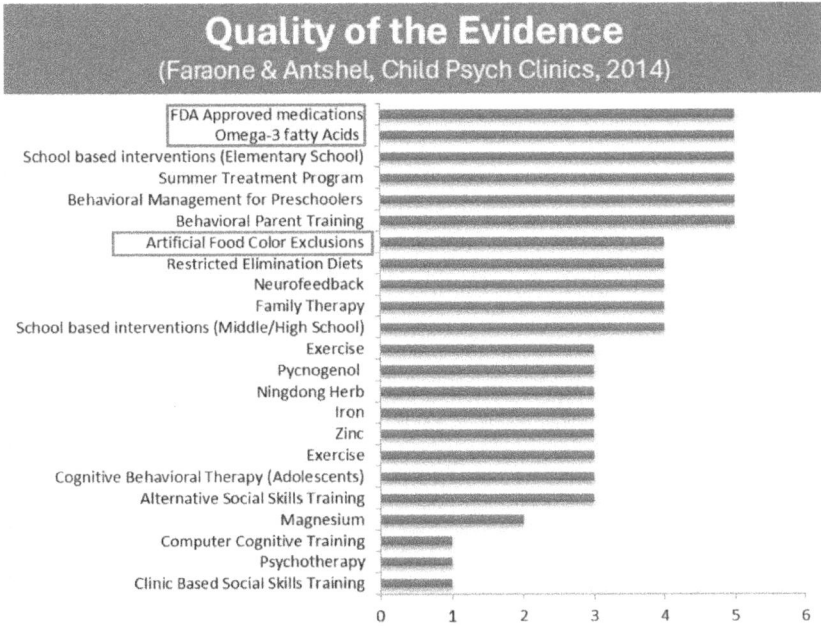

Figure 4. Stephen V. Faraone, "Quality of ADHD Treatments" *An Overview of Attention Deficit Hyperactivity Disorder* (2022): 35, https://www.adhdevidence.org/resources#slides.

of treating their ADHD with stimulants. Eighty-five percent of the time, either amphetamine or methylphenidate will greatly improve the person's life. Further micronutrient support will help the medications work better and may address some underlying imbalances that are not addressed by drugs alone. See Figures 4 and 5 for a list of treatments listed by efficacy.

"I was so frustrated after both Ritalin and Adderall failed and made me more irritable and anxious. I was hoping for the same quick fix my friends with ADHD got when they started on their medications. Fortunately, we dug deeper and discovered that my vitamin D, cholesterol, and thyroid were all off.

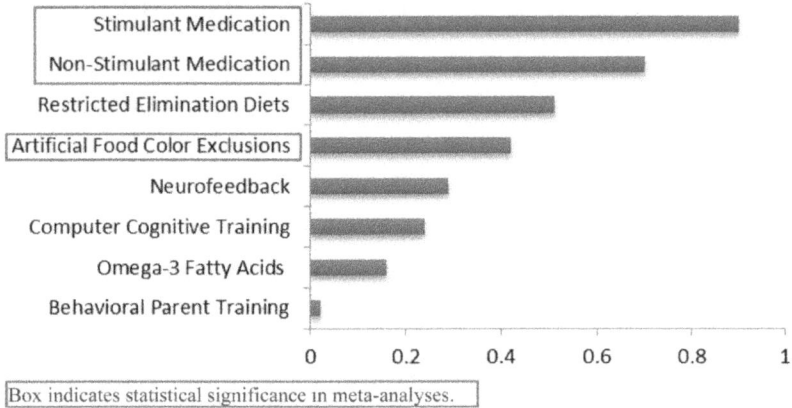

Figure 5. Faraone, "Magnitude of Treatment Effect," *An Overview of Attention Deficit Hyperactivity Disorder:* 36.

Also, I had MTHFR deficiency and needed L-methylfolate. After six months of addressing these deficiencies, I slept more, had increased energy, could concentrate better, and my mood was 100 percent improved. The best part was my kids and husband said they had their mama and wife back."

"Even though my ADHD got better after treating it with Adderall, my mood only improved a bit. Once I started taking vitamins and cut gluten out of my diet, I found that I was no longer depressed four out of seven days. I had no idea that a low cholesterol level would be bad for me and that zinc mattered at all."

CHAPTER 7 PEARLS

1. Micronutrient imbalances can be a root cause of many mental health problems.

2. Assessment from a battery of routine blood, urine, and hair tests can be used to improve key vitamins, minerals, and neurotransmitters.

3. Most providers are unfamiliar with doing laboratory and genetic testing and may need support in learning what to order and how to interpret the results.

4. Stimulant medications are effective 85 percent of the time and will work better when other micronutrient imbalances are also addressed.

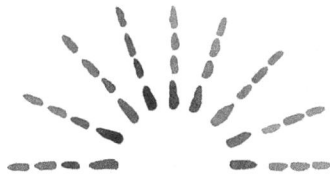

CHAPTER 8

Medications

I needed to update you on something incredible. Today's dosage was 15 mg in the morning and 15 mg in the afternoon. The results were absolutely astounding. Up until now, I noticed some difference in my concentration during the day, but the big difference was that I had energy at the end of the day to play with my kids like I hadn't had in years. I used to curl up in a ball on my bed at the end of the day because I was so fatigued from all of the decisions and work that I had to do, to try to do something with my kiddos felt like I was fighting against my will, and I had no willpower to overcome it, and so I would just basically be under the covers wanting the world to leave me alone. And I felt so bad about myself because I wanted to be a good dad and felt like it was all passing me by without my engagement. I felt ashamed of myself.

With the more normalized energy at the end of the day, I've been much more engaged with my kids, and it hasn't felt like a burden to do it; it's just been natural and fun. In the past, doing stuff with them, I would force myself to do things, but I wasn't very present or engaged—it was like I was making myself walk through the motions of doing things with them, but I really wasn't enjoying it. I was doing things that I thought I should do but never felt very present. The last couple weeks, that has been completely different; doing things with them feels natural and fun, and it's not like I even feel like I'm making some big decision to play with them. I'm just doing it naturally, and it does not feel burdensome. Turns out I really like my kids. I've been playing catch with my daughter and played chess yesterday with my son and was really enjoying engaging in conversations with both of them—it just felt so natural and easy.

So, the energy at the end of the day has been really exciting to me, but today was the first day I really noticed the impact of the ability to concentrate. I had a project on my desk that I have been procrastinating on for five and a half months. In my other previous state of mind, it felt like this incredibly burdensome, tedious, boring, and difficult project that I would have to spend three to four hours slogging through drudgery to try to get done. Today, not only did I do that project, but it was done in 20 minutes! It's like my brain can quickly see the connections and what needs to be done and then simply do it without feeling like it's some sort of impossible task. And there is nothing "high" about my state of mind; quite the contrary. I feel calm, engaged, and focused. I used to think I was the dumb one of my family, but today I actually felt smart.

I feel like the results with me have been so remarkably similar to the impact that it had on that first patient of yours that you described to me. I really feel like a miracle is taking place with me, and I am so very thankful, Maggie. In the past there's no way I would've been able to write an email at the end of the day like this, but now it's easy. I am so grateful to you, and very excited about continuing to work with you! A very big thank you and a hug!

When one hits the nail on the head, like this client did, it is because the right drug, dosage, and length of coverage are perfectly achieved. Once ADHD has been diagnosed, how do we address this condition? I advise starting with education, learning about what it is and what it is not. The National Attention Deficit Hyperactivity Disorder website (www.add.org) is an excellent place to start. I also recommend Jessica McCabe's YouTube channel "How to ADHD" and her book with the same title. There are many good books; please check the reference list at the back of this one for my favorite authors and resources.

Once you have a basic understanding of ADHD and you believe you may have the condition, download the ADHD ASRS form, do a quick self-assessment, and see your local ADHD specialist for an official diagnosis. I recommend starting on stimulant medications as soon as possible. There is no advantage to trying an antidepressant first. Many providers were educated to treat anxiety and depression before prescribing stimulants. As I've mentioned previously, ADHD is very often the underlying cause of anxiety and depression. If you are still anxious or depressed after proper treatment of your ADHD, then ask your provider for additional treatment.

"At times, medication has caused some friction in my relationship with my partner. However, this has only been when the balance isn't quite right, and I have found myself

struggling with irritability or apathy as a result of the medication wearing off, which helped me realize I need to take enough to cover the full day. The big picture is that I feel it has helped improve my relationships by helping me achieve better reliability, organizational skills, and more focus within my relationship with my partner. Oddly, my mood started improving too. Maybe getting things done and sleeping more made me feel better."

CAUSES OF ADHD

While the research is ongoing, some things are clear: ADHD is not caused by poor parenting, family problems, ineffective teachers or schools, too much TV, or online activities. Greenblatt indicates that multiple variables—including diet; mineral, vitamin, amino acid, and other deficiencies; and environmental toxins—significantly contribute to symptoms of ADHD and, of course, all other mental health conditions.[41] We know that there are decreases in neurotransmitters—norepinephrine and dopamine—in the prefrontal lobes of the cortex of the brain. Positron emission tomography (PET scan) shows a link between a person's ability to pay attention and the level of activity in the brain. In people with ADHD, the brain areas that control attention used less glucose, indicating those areas were less active.

ADHD runs in families—there is a 25 to 35 percent probability that parents with ADHD will pass it on to their children. Even if not diagnosed, you may know of a relative who was described as disruptive or had too much energy or was a ne'er-do-well. These could be signs of undiagnosed ADHD.

---

[41] U.S. CDC, "About Attention-Deficit/Hyperactivity Disorder (ADHD)."

When environmental and biochemical stressors are addressed, medications may become optional for some people. However, for most people living with ADHD, medications will make the difference between barely getting by much of the time and thriving most of the time.

In my experience, the proper use of stimulant medications is life-changing, and I'm eager for you to learn about the simple guidelines you can bring to your prescriber to increase your odds of finding a life-changing experience. Again, broccoli, love, and exercise are great adjuncts but are, in themselves, inadequate to treat brains that need more dopamine and norepinephrine. Once treated, you will be more able to improve your diet and address any micronutrient deficiencies that are contributing to your symptoms. Some people can stop taking stimulants, but most will continue to use them for the rest of their lives.

NATIONAL PRACTICE TREATMENT GUIDELINES

The United States is still working on creating national guidelines for treating adults with ADHD, so I have drawn from guidelines from the United Kingdom's National Institute for Health and Care Excellence (NICE),[42] the Canadian ADHD Resource Alliance (CADDRA),[43] the Australian ADHD Professional Association (AADPA),[44] and the American Academy of Family Practice

---

[42] National Institute for Health and Care Excellence (NICE), "Attention deficit hyperactivity disorder: diagnosis and management," *NICE Guideline NG87* (updated 2019), https://www.nice.org.uk/guidance/ng87.

[43] Canada ADHD Resource Alliance (CADDRA), *Canadian ADHD Practice Guidelines, Third Edition* (CADDRA, 2011), https://caddra.ca/pdfs/caddraGuidelines2011.pdf.

[44] Australian ADHD Professionals Association (AADPA), *Australian Evidence-Based Clinical Practice Guideline for Attention Deficit Hyperactivity Disorder (ADHD)* (2022), https://aadpa.com.au/guideline/.

(AAFP), which offers guidelines for children and adolescents.[45] Finally, Faraone, president of the World Federation of ADHD, is on the special committee of the American Professional Society of ADHD and Related Disorders (APSARD) to lead the development of United States adult ADHD guidelines. He also founded the ADHD Evidence Project, which contributes to making evidence-based recommendations available to professionals and the public.[46]

INTRODUCTION TO STIMULANTS

Stimulant medications, including amphetamines (e.g., Adderall, Adderall XR, Vyvanse, Dexedrine, MyDayis) and methylphenidate (e.g., Ritalin, Concerta, Focalin, JornayPM) have a calming and focusing effect on individuals with ADHD. They are prescribed for daily extended use and come in the form of tablets, capsules, patches, and liquid preparations of varying dosages. Treatment with stimulants, often in conjunction with micronutrients and psychotherapy, helps improve ADHD symptoms and the person's self-esteem, thinking ability, and social and family interactions. Scientific literature, the American Academy of Pediatrics, the American Academy of Child and Adolescent Psychiatry, the AAFP, and the American Psychiatric Association consider these medicines to be the best treatment options for children, adolescents, and adults. Finally, the dosage of medications has no relationship to the person's age, sex, or weight.

---

[45] American Academy of Family Practice, *ADHD in Children and Adolescents* (2020), https://www.aafp.org/family-physician/patient-care/clinical-recommendations/all-clinical-recommendations/ADHD.html.

[46] The ADHD Evidence Project, accessed June 5, 2025, https://www.adhdevidence.org/.

HOW STIMULANTS WORK

Stimulants don't work by increasing stimulation; rather, they increase the neurotransmitters dopamine and nor-epinephrine. There are two types of stimulants: methylphenidate (Ritalin) and amphetamines (Adderall). All other ADHD stimulant medications contain some derivative of these two core ingredients.

dopamine
A neurotransmitter that elevates mood, increases the ability to attend, and facilitates learning.

norepinephrine
A neurotransmitter that impacts ability to focus and attend, memory, and sleep/wake cycles.

In addition to Ritalin and Adderall, the nonstimulants atomoxetine (Strattera) and viloxazine (Qelbree) also raise dopamine and norepineph-rine. Also, two blood pressure medications, clonidine (Kapvay) and guanfacine (Intuniv), raise norepinephrine.

INTERNATIONAL RECOMMENDATIONS FOR TREATING ADHD[47]

AADPA created comprehensive practice guidelines in 2022. I recommend reading the guidelines (see the reference section at the back of this book). Some key takeaways:

1. Use medicine and non-pharmacological treatment (e.g., lifestyle, therapy, coaching, behavioral support).

---

[47] AADPA Guidelines, 2022, 93–98.

2. Children under five should be assessed by a clinician and offered non-pharmacological interventions.

3. Children and adults may be offered methylphenidate (Ritalin), dexamphetamine (Adderall), or lisdexamfetamine (Vyvanse), an amphetamine derivative.

4. The guidelines recommend the same prescription advice for adults over 65, with careful monitoring for side effects.

5. The clinician and family should decide which type, dose, and formulation is best to begin with.

6. Nonstimulants atomoxetine (Strattera), guanfacine (Intuniv), clonidine (Kapvay), or viloxazine (Qelbree) should be offered to children and adolescents if:

   a. stimulants are contraindicated;

   b. the person cannot tolerate methylphenidate, dexamphetamine, or lisdexamfetamine;

   c. symptoms have not responded to separate trials of methylphenidate, dexamphetamine, or lisdexamfetamine at adequate doses; or

   d. the clinician believes the medication may be a beneficial adjunct to the current regimen.

7. Second-line treatments for adults with ADHD can be offered: bupropion, clonidine, modafinil, or venlafaxine.

8. Be aware of the risks of appetite suppression for people with disordered eating.

9. Short- and long-acting stimulants may be offered together to optimize effect.

10. Drug holidays are not recommended (NICE guidelines).

11. Find a way to support a person with ADHD's adherence to taking medications. This can include pill boxes, schedules, timers, reducing barriers at pharmacies, and ensuring prescribers are up to date with monthly prescriptions.

> **NICE guidelines**
> Evidence-based recommendations for health and social care in England and Wales, developed by the National Institute for Health and Care Excellence (NICE).

CLINICAL RECOMMENDATIONS FROM MY PRACTICE

☀ I prefer to seek precise dosing by starting with a short-acting tablet that can be carefully titrated and then converting to an equivalent long-acting version. Be sure to cover all 12–16 hours the person is awake.

- I strongly recommend combining short- and long-acting stimulants and often suggest that my clients cover the 12+ hours with a "sandwich approach" of short-acting, followed 3 hours later with extended release, and then topped off with another short-acting, especially when taking Adderall XR.

- For example: 7 a.m. Adderall IR 10 mg; 10 a.m. Adderall XR 20 mg; and 4–6 p.m. Adderall IR 10 mg. (See Figure 7 for more on page 96.)

☀ My experience indicates that atomoxetine is rarely effective, although I have seen some autistic clients benefit from it.

☀ In my observation, the efficacy of nonstimulant medications pales in contrast to stimulants.

☀ Guanfacine and clonidine address mood dys-regulation (see Chapter 5). They improve attention by decreasing the distracting mental back-ground "noise."

☀ Prior recreational drug users have been shown to use illicit drugs less when they maintain their prop-erly prescribed stimulants.

☀ A 90-day mail order prescription, if available, can greatly enhance adherence and access.

Dopamine and norepinephrine are associated with plea-sure, movement, and attention. Improving access will heighten focus and help people be in a better mood and want to be more active. The therapeutic effect of stimulants is achieved by a dos-age that starts low and is increased gradually, resulting in slow and steady increases of dopamine and norepinephrine.

One way to understand the proper use of stimulants is to equate them to using the perfect eyeglass prescription. Imag-ine having trouble reading because you have vision problems or can't focus. Your provider says, "Let's have you try wearing glasses" and you put on a pair of 1.25 reading glasses. You notice that things are a bit clearer, then you increase to 1.5 and they are much clearer, so you keep going. 1.75 is really great and 2.0 seems crystal clear, but then you try 2.25 lenses, and, although you can read much better than without glasses, you have a bit of a headache, and things are a little blurry. When you try the 2.5 reading glasses, your eyes hurt, and you take them off and say, "I'd rather not use these."

This is analogous to how stimulant medications work. If you start at the low dose of 5 mg of methylphenidate (Ritalin) or mixed amphetamines (Adderall) and increase by 2.5 mg per dose every other day, within a week or two, you'll reach the ideal therapeutic dose. Once you go beyond the ideal dose, you'll have some mild side effects, like anxiety, or the return of brain fog or possibly hyperfocus on the wrong thing. This is the indication that yesterday's dose was your actual ideal therapeutic dose. Once the correct dose has been determined, you can convert the short-acting dose into an extended-release version. Generally, the extended-release amphetamine will be twice the dosage of the immediate-release, so for a 10 mg dose, the equivalent extended-release capsule would be 20 mg of mixed amphetamine. Ritalin is more complicated, as the long-acting equivalent, Concerta, is calculated differently: 10 mg of IR Ritalin equates to about 36 mg of long-acting Concerta or methylphenidate ER. Consult with your practitioner about prescribing the correct amounts and discuss the idea of "wearing your glasses while you are awake and needing to focus."

Faraone confirms that methylphenidate (Ritalin) improves emotional dysregulation, executive functioning, and intellectual disability. Furthermore, stimulants reduce anxiety, aggression, the risk of suicide, and psychotic events. There is also no risk of adverse cardiac events.[48]

Dodson evaluated his patients' response using the Test of Variables of Attention (TOVA), a 27-minute computerized test assessing attention, impulsiveness, and reaction time—three

---

[48] Le Zhang et al., "Risk of Cardiovascular Diseases Associated With Medications Used in Attention-Deficit/Hyperactivity Disorder: A Systematic Review and Meta-analysis," *JAMA Network Open*, 5(11) (2022), https://doi.org/10.1001/jamanetworkopen.2022.43597.

common characteristics compromised in those with ADHD.[49] He found that the dose of medication that helps people with ADHD function within the normal reference range is very specific. The graphic depiction of this (see Figure 6) shows not a bell-shaped curve but a sharp peak. As with eyeglasses, there is one dose, and one dose only, that will help any individual focus most clearly—not a range. Secondly, this clarity is achieved with only one of the two stimulants, amphetamine (Adderall) or methylphenidate (Ritalin). Dodson offered his patients a two-week trial of each stimulant class to learn which drug worked best for them.

In the following graph, you can see that this person's ideal dose is about 12.5 mg of stimulant, and that even at 15 mg, and certainly by 17.5 mg, they have fallen outside of the normal reference range and unfortunately have side effects. These can include increased blood pressure, headaches, dry mouth, jaw-clenching, irritability, and anxiety. However, decreasing the dose back down to the previous day's dose yields what I call the "Magic Mountain" dose (in reference to the obvious ideal peak in the graph); the person will feel calm and focused. Their side effects go away, and 60 percent of people taking stimulants will sleep better on them. When they go just 2.5 mg too high, they "fall off the mountain" and have the side effects described above. It's necessary to experience "falling off the mountain" to be certain of the ideal dose. Without it, you risk settling for a "nearly there" dose and possibly being under-prescribed by as much as 20 percent.

[49] TOVA.com, accessed July 15, 2025, https://tovatest.com/.

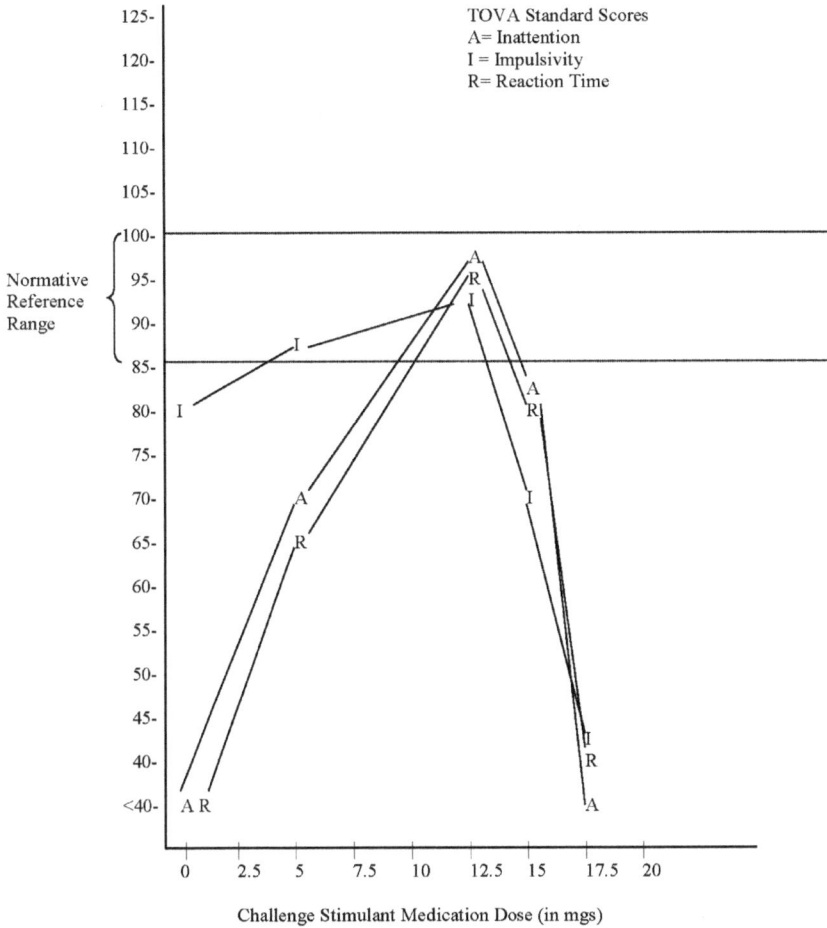

Figure 6. Finding the "Magic Mountain" in Dosing Amounts.

KEY POINTS ABOUT HOW TO USE STIMULANT MEDICATIONS

Unfortunately, many people are given a standard starting dose of 10 mg of Adderall or Ritalin and never realize that they need 12.5 mg, or worse, 15 mg. Consequently, they "see" better but not quite clearly. Just a slight increase in prescription can offer a significant improvement in focus. Conversely, if they only need 7.5 mg, they are living with side effects, similar to wearing a prescription lens that is a little too strong. Consequently, they are less likely to use their medication regularly because of the irritability or headache they experience. This happened to my client "Matt," whom I described previously. Part of why he didn't go back to his senior-year Adderall prescription was because he felt irritable when taking it. Decades later, when he tried Concerta (long-acting Ritalin), he found the perfect medication, dose, and length of action. How we wish he had not endured so many years of underperforming and suicidal depression.

This is why it is critical *not* to start with a standard starting dose of 10 mg of Adderall or Ritalin, as only about 40 to 50 percent of people fall into this range. Ten percent of my clients need less than this standard dose, and 40 percent require more than the Federal Drug Administration's (FDA) recommended 40 to 60 mg per day guidelines. Under the guidance of a skilled professional, a proper choice of medication and dose is possible.

Once you've determined your exact dosage, the goal is to medicate to address the hours that you are awake and need to focus. Imagine if you could only wear your glasses in school, or in the morning, or when you have more difficult tasks to complete. People with ADHD, just like the rest of the population, need to focus all day long. There are various ways to accomplish this, and, unfortunately, since several of the extended-release versions of methylphenidate and amphetamines are quite expensive, the general recommendation is to start with the most basic generic version of short-acting Ritalin and Adderall. Many providers prefer to begin with a long-acting (extended-release) version of the medication because these are more difficult to abuse and cover 6 to 12 hours, in comparison with the 4 hours for which a tablet of Ritalin or Adderall will be active.

It is much more difficult to titrate the extended-release capsule versions, which generally can't be divided. For this reason, I suggest starting with immediate-release tablets that can be carefully titrated to the ideal dose. Once the right dosage has been determined, then you can add an extended release. Unfortunately, long-acting Adderall capsules only last about six hours. Concerta, long-acting Ritalin, lasts 8 to 10 hours for most people, and Vyvanse, an amphetamine, lasts 6 to 12 hours.

Many providers give their clients an extended-release formulation first thing in the morning. These long-acting medications take 60 to 90 minutes to activate. This can be problematic when an individual has a hard time getting going in the morning. Generally, people with ADHD have sleep issues and are not morning people. Even if your prescriber offers you a short-acting booster tablet in the afternoon, you will find that the drop-off can be quite sudden, leaving you feeling tired, possibly irritable, and unable to focus on much once the medication has worn off.

To address this issue, I recommend taking an immediate-release tablet first thing in the morning and then about three hours later taking the extended-release version of the same medication. Occasionally the length of action of the extended-release amphetamine Vyvanse is long enough to cover the full 12 hours, and people will not need to supplement with immediate-release Adderall. Most of the time my clients find they prefer to start the day with the "kick in the pants" immediate-release tablet. The pills take a modest 20 to 30 minutes to activate. This is followed three hours later by the extended release that takes one to one and a half hours to start working. The extended release also has a much slower discontinuation, or drop-off period, creating a gentler descent and enabling people to remain focused in the late afternoon and sometimes into the evening hours. See Figure 7 for an example of the 'Sandwich' approach to using short and long acting stimulants.

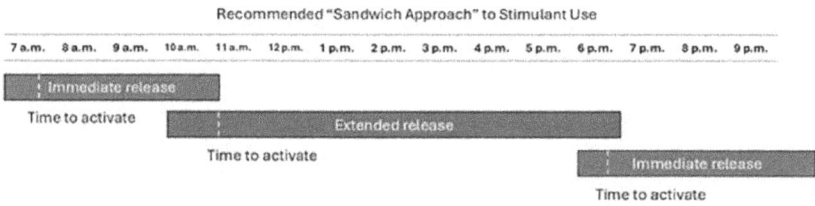

Recommended "Sandwich Approach" to Stimulant Use

Figure 7. Recommended approach to stimulant use.

Many of my clients also find they benefit from my "sandwich" protocol: a short-acting tablet first thing in the morning, followed three hours later by an extended-release, and then about 6 to 8 hours later, a second short-acting tablet. This works well for people who need to be able to stay focused in the evening hours, such as parents, students, adults with 12-hour shifts, and those with evening hobbies.

Again, these medications are not dependent on your sex, age, or weight. Remember Matt, my six foot two, 220-pound client who was on the lowest dose of long-acting Ritalin? He's still on that dose, because, in terms of Ritalin, he is a lightweight. He needed the lowest possible prescription. Just like eyeglasses, it depends on the individual. I have 110-pound women who are taking two extended-release Vyvanse per day and some men who are on just 5 mg of Adderall a day.

SUMMARY AND FINAL CONSIDERATIONS

Determine if amphetamine or methylphenidate works best for you. If you've never tried either, no one in your family is taking one of these meds, and you are over age 15, start with amphetamines. Once you know the dose that is right for you, replace the second short-acting tablet with an extended-release version of the same medication. If you require a third dose later in the afternoon or evening, use the same dose you used in the morning (just like glasses), and experiment with it on a weekend in case you are one of the 40 percent of people whose sleep will be disturbed by late-afternoon stimulants. If the first stimulant you try doesn't feel right and causes side effects, you will know this within a few days to a couple of weeks. Don't keep trying it—switch to the other stimulant and start back at 5 mg twice a day. Repeat the slow titration up the "magic mountain" until you reach the descent on the other side of the peak, as experienced by the introduction of a side effect and "fall off." Then return to the previous day's dose, 2.5 mg less than when you had the side effect.

Once you have determined your proper dose, it is very rare that this dose will change. People generally do not build up a tolerance and may be on the same dose for years. Generally, individuals who find that their meds "stopped working" have changed brands, were on the wrong dose in the first place, started taking high levels of citric acid (which breaks down amphetamines), or may have some other significant GI issue that interferes with the absorption of the extended-release version of the medication.

> *"After I reached the correct dose of Adderall, it was like a giant weight lifted from me. Suddenly I could move more easily throughout my day. Everything felt clearer and easier to complete. I didn't feel jacked; I just felt focused, like myself when I'm doing something I enjoy. It was amazing. I just wish they didn't wear off after four hours. I can't wait to try the long-acting ones."*

> *"My husband noticed that I was listening to him better and didn't keep asking him to repeat himself and for the first time in years, I only went back to the house once instead of five times to get things before I drove off."*

> *"I don't know why, but my mood was much better, I felt genuinely happier and hopeful that I'd actually be able to reach my*

goals and make something of my life. Honestly, this is so much better than Prozac and all those times when I just tried harder."

"Be open to using medication and to think of it no differently than you would think of someone who needs to take medication for other things such as diabetes. Understand that medication is not the end-all in the process of treating ADHD. It's one piece of the treatment process that when put together with other pieces makes it possible for you to function and feel differently about yourself."

MEDICATION NAMES AND PRESCRIBING PRACTICES

There is a lack of clear recommendations for professionals and the public since national guidelines have yet to be established in the US. ADHD Evidence has produced helpful charts summarizing what medications are available, see Figures 8 and 9 and Tables 3 through 8 for lists of medications and appropriate dosage recommendations

Medications Approved by FDA for ADHD

• FDA Approved Stimulants (DAT reuptake inhibitors)
  – Methylphenidate & Amphetamine
  – IR & ER formulations
  – Duration range 4 to 16 hours
  – Liquid and chewable forms available
• FDA Approved Non-Stimulants
  – Atomoxetine (NET reuptake inhibitor)
  – Extended Release Viloxazine (NET & DAT reuptake inhibitor)
  – Alpha-2 Agonists
    • Extended Release Guanfacine
    • Extended Release Clonidine

Slide courtesy of www.ADHDevidence.org

Figure 8. Medications Approved by the FDA for ADHD. Faraone, *An Overview of ADHD*, 40.

Medications Not Approved by FDA for ADHD But Used Off-Label

- Bupropion
- Tricyclic Anti-depressants
- Modafinil
- Memantine

Slide courtesy of www.ADHDevidence.org

Figure 9. Medications Not Approved by the FDA for ADHD but Used Off-Label. Faraone, *An Overview of ADHD*, 41.

DEXTROAMPHETAMINE AND AMPHETAMINE (MIXED SALTS)					
SHORT-ACTING	ONSET	DURATION	INITIAL DOSAGE	TITRATION	MAINTENANCE DOSE
Adderall and generic equivalents	30 min	4–6 hours	5 mg once to thrice per day	Increase daily dose 2.5 mg/ dose every 2 days	5–90 mg per day in 2–3 divided doses
Long-acting					
Adderall XR and generic equivalents	>1 hour	6–10 hours	10 mg once per day	Increase daily dose by 5 mg at 2-day intervals	10–60 mg once per day

Table 3. Dosing Recommendations.

METHYLPHENIDATE					
SHORT-ACTING	**ONSET**	**DURATION**	**INITIAL DOSAGE**	**TITRATION**	**MAINTENANCE DOSE**
Ritalin and generic equivalents	30 min; delayed if taken with high-fat meal	3–5 hours	5 mg once to thrice per day before breakfast and lunch	Increase daily dose by 2.5 mg/dose every 2 days	5–60 mg per day in 2 or 3 divided doses
Long-acting					
Concerta and generic equivalents	1 hour; plateau at 1–4 hours; peak at 6 hours after dose	8–12 hours	18 mg once per day in morning	Increase daily dose to 27, 36, 54, and 72 mg, until a side effect is noted	18–72 mg once per day

Table 4. Dosing Recommendations.

METHYLPHENIDATES SHORT-ACTING/IMMEDIATE RELEASE	
BRAND	**GENERIC**
Ritalin	Methylphenidate
Focalin	Dexmethylphenidate

Table 5. Methylphenidates, Short-acting/Immediate release.

METHYLPHENIDATES LONG-ACTING/EXTENDED RELEASE	
BRAND	**GENERIC**
Concerta	Methylphenidate ER
Ritalin SR	Methylphenidate SR
Ritalin LA	Methylphenidate LA
Metadate CD	Methylphenidate CD
Focalin XR	Dexmethylphenidate XR
QuilliChew ER	
Quillivant XR	
Aztarys	
Jornay PM	
Cotempla XR-ODT	
Daytrana (transdermal)	
Relexxii	
Apentsio XR	

Table 6. Methylphenidates, Long-acting/Extended release.

AMPHETAMINES SHORT-ACTING/IMMEDIATE RELEASE	
MIXED AMPHETAMINE SALTS	**DEXTROAMPHETAMINE**
Adderall	ProCentra
Evekeo	Zenzedi
Evekeo ODT	

Table 7. Amphetamines, Short-acting/Immediate release.

AMPHETAMINES			
LONG-ACTING/EXTENDED RELEASE			
MIXED AMPHETAMINE SALTS		**DEXAMPHETAMINES**	
BRAND	**GENERIC**	**BRAND**	**GENERIC**
Adderall XR (capsule)	Dextroamphetamine-amphetamine XR	Vyvance (capsule or chewable)	Lisdexamphetamine
Adzenys ER (liquid)	Amphetamine	Xelstrym (transdermal)	Dextroamphetamine
Adzenys XR ODT (dissolvable)	Dextroamphetamine-amphetamine XR	ProCentra	Dextroamphetamine sulfate
Dyanavel XR (liquid or chewable)	Amphetamine	Dexedrine	Dextroamphetamine sulfate
Mydayis (capsule)	Dextroamphetamine-amphetamine XR		

Table 8. Amphetamines, Long-acting/Extended release.

EFFECTIVENESS

The National Institute of Mental Health (NIMH) began a large treatment study in 1992.[50] Data from this 14-month study showed that stimulant medication is the most effective treatment for ADHD, as long as it is administered in doses adjusted for each child to give the best response—either alone or in

---

[50] MTA Cooperative Group, "A 14-Month Randomized Clinical Trial of Treatment Strategies for Attention-Deficit/Hyperactivity Disorder," *Archives of General Psychiatry—JAMA Network*, 56(12) (1999): 1073–1086, https://doi.org/10.1001/archpsyc.56.12.1073.

combination with behavioral therapy, in contrast to behavioral therapy alone.

While medicine alone is a proven treatment for ADHD, the Multimodal Treatment of ADHD study (MTA study) found that combining behavioral treatment with medicine was useful in helping families, teachers, and children learn ways to manage and modify the behaviors that cause problems at home and school.

Though not a cure, medication treatment does allow the person to function better, manage their ADHD, and benefit from academic and related interventions intended to improve their overall functioning in school, at home, at work, and in the community. A percentage of children may no longer require treatment as they grow into late adolescence and adulthood. Again, "pills don't build skills." Although in my experience, stimulants are incredibly effective for 90 percent of people diagnosed with ADHD, it is also important to develop strategies and learning techniques to help build systems that support your "interest-based nervous system."

SIDE EFFECTS

Any medication can produce unwanted side effects. Common and predictable side effects from stimulant medication include reduced appetite, weight loss, problems sleeping, dry mouth, headaches, dizziness, upset stomach, or mild diarrhea. These can usually be managed by reducing the dose, changing the type of delivery (immediate-acting tablet or long-acting capsule), changing the time administered, switching to another medication, and addressing underlying vitamin and mineral deficiencies.

SAFETY

Interactions with ADHD medications do exist. It is important to tell your provider and pharmacist about all over-the-counter (OTC) and prescription medications, herbal supplements, decongestants, caffeinated products, and vitamins you are taking. Additionally, speak to your provider and pharmacist before you take a new medication or supplement. Before starting stimulant therapy, talk to your provider if you have high blood pressure, heart abnormalities, mood or anxiety disorders, motor tics (sudden, involuntary movements), or Tourette's syndrome; are using a medication that is a monoamine oxidase inhibitor (MAOI); have a history of seizures; or are considering pregnancy.

PRESCRIPTIONS

schedule 2 (II) drug
A drug with an accepted medical use for treatment in the US but which may have a high potential for abuse or dependency.

Since the Drug Enforcement Administration (DEA) has classified stimulants as Schedule 2 medications that have the potential for abuse, they require strict control compared to other medications. Providers who prescribe stimulants must register with the DEA and refills cannot be routinely ordered via phone or fax. Prescriptions can only be written for three months at a time without refills. Generally, three-month scripts can only be obtained from mail-order pharmacies, and most local pharmacies will only fill one month at a time. Costs of medications, both brand name and generics, vary greatly depending on insurance coverage and pharmacies. To avoid medication that is too expensive, discuss medication costs with the prescribing provider. If you have insurance, many companies will require your provider submit a "prior authorization" confirming they will cover this medication. Prior authorizations may also be required by insurance companies for any increase in dose. This can take several days to complete.

FREQUENTLY ASKED QUESTIONS: MEDICATIONS

How do I know if the medication is working?

If the dose of stimulant medication is adjusted for best effect, you will see beneficial effects within 30 to 90 minutes, depending on the dose and formulation used. When it is working, many ADHD symptoms will lessen in severity.

Common signs that medication is working

Sustained focus: You may be able to focus for longer periods of time than you can without medications; not hyperfocus, just calm, sustained focus that you can direct and helps you be more productive. Once you get started on a boring task, you can maintain attention longer.

Hyperactivity/restlessness: You will exhibit fewer signs of hyperactivity: fidgeting, twirling hair, picking nails, shifting in seat, fast thoughts, "brain chatter," or the urge to walk during times you are expected to stay still, such as standing in line, watching a movie, and sitting through class.

Decreased impulsivity: You should have less impulsivity, both physical and verbal: interrupting people less, getting out of your seat less often, and fewer impulsive thoughts.

Improved mood: At the optimal dose of medication, people often report overall improved mood, less anxiety, lower stress (often related to higher productivity), and fewer social challenges.

Greater attention to detail: You should be able to complete a form without skipping a line and may catch small mistakes before they happen.

Better memory: You'll be better able to remember names, not need to reread a page of a book, and not ask people to repeat instructions.

Better sleep: The right medication helps children and adults with ADHD fall asleep by slowing down their brains enough to quiet the racing thoughts that previously kept them awake. You may feel more alert when you wake in the morning.

What happens if I miss my dose?

If you miss a dose of your medication, take it as soon as you remember, if it is not too close to when your next dose is due; discuss this with your health-care provider. If it is close to your next dose, take the next dose and skip the missed dose. Do not double your next dose or take more than what you have been told to take. Taking a dose too close to bedtime may hinder your ability to fall asleep, for 40% of people.

> *"When I first started seeing Maggie, I had 10 episodes of being hospitalized for alcohol abuse. I blacked out regularly. My life was a wreck, and my parents were ready to give up on me. She recognized my ADHD, treated me with high doses of amphetamines, and required me to do a rehab program*

that included AA and weekly check-ins with an alcohol coun-selor. I've been sober for two years and have held down a full-time job. Stimulants literally saved my life. When I feel the craving, I know to take a little more medication in the late afternoon. I finally have some hope that I can find hap-piness again."

Will using stimulants increase my chances of misusing illegal drugs?

It is a popular misconception that using stimulants may lead to their abuse. People with ADHD who have tried cocaine or methamphetamine found that they often felt calmer, rather than high, when using these drugs. If a person tends to try to quiet their racing, often self-critical mind by drinking or using cannabis or other drugs, having them take an additional dose of their prescribed stimulant can often decrease or remove the craving completely.

Pharmacological treatment of ADHD in individuals with severe substance use disorder may decrease the risk of relapse and increase these patients' ability to follow a non-pharmacological rehabilitation plan, thereby improving their long-term out-comes.[51] In a 2011 study, it was found that stimulant use did not make drug use worse.[52] In my clinical practice, my clients

---

[51] Berit Bihlar Muld, et al., "Long-Term Outcomes of Pharmacologically Treated Versus Non-Treated Adults with ADHD and Substance Use Disorder: A Naturalistic Study," *Journal of Substance Abuse Treatment*, 51 (2014): 82–90, https://doi.org/10.1016/j.jsat.2014.11.005.

[52] Paula Riggs, et al., "Randomized Controlled Trial of Osmotic-Release Methylphenidate With Cognitive-Behavioral Therapy in Adolescents With Attention-Deficit/Hyperactivity Disorder and Substance Use Disorders," *Journal of the American Academy of Child & Adolescent Psychiatry*, 50(9) (2011): 903–914, https://doi.org/10.1016/j.jaac.2011.06.010.

who have struggled with drug or alcohol use generally decrease, or even stop, "self-medicating" with alcohol or drugs once they receive the correct stimulant, dose, and duration of coverage. This is where taking it all day long really makes a big difference.

Are methylphenidate and amphetamine the same as meth?

Although amphetamine medications *sound* like meth (meth-amphetamine), there are many important differences, starting with a bit of chemistry. In the simplest terms, amphetamine lacks an extra structural component, allowing it to be more therapeutic and safer to prescribe. Although methamphetamine and amphetamines can have similar stimulant effects, meth's effects are longer lasting and toxic. The extra structural component enables meth to better penetrate the blood-brain barrier and causes it to have more addictive properties compared to amphetamine medications. Amphetamine medications have also been around since the 1920s, allowing research to create safe and effective guidelines for use as a treatment for ADHD.

Does the use of stimulants make a person more vulnerable to drug or alcohol addiction later?

Concerns have been raised that stimulants prescribed to treat a child's or adolescent's ADHD could affect an individual's vulnerability to developing later drug problems—either by increasing the risk or by providing a degree of protection. The studies conducted so far have found no differences in later substance use for children with ADHD who received treatment and those who did not. This suggests treatment with ADHD medication appears not to affect an individual's risk for developing a substance use disorder.

"Ask your body what you need. I used to just take my meds at the same time every day without thinking much about it. Which was fine when I was very busy with school or work and needed energy and consistency. But sometimes I'll take my next dose at the 'scheduled' time without noticing that my brain is still working off my last dose. Taking more Ritalin, for me, doesn't make me more focused or productive; instead, I feel tired and weighed down, when I take it too soon."

When does my medicine need to be adjusted?

If you are experiencing side effects—headache, nausea, irritability, dry mouth, reduced appetite, problems sleeping, headache, upset stomach, or mild diarrhea—your dosage is either the wrong stimulant, too high a dose, or taken too late in the day. Review the pharmacy drug information provided with your prescription for specific drug side effects and report any that you experience to your provider.

What about weekends and drug holidays?

Think about wearing your glasses. Would you take them off on the weekends or holidays? There is no benefit in not taking your medication, only disadvantages. If you sleep in, you can skip a dose, but I do not recommend skipping a full day. People do not tend to build up tolerance. If you hear of this happening, it is probably because that person's dosage is too high. They are on the wrong side of the "magic mountain" and are overstimulated.

They should go down by 10 to 20 percent and see if the side effects abate.

Why did my medicine stop working or suddenly give me side effects?

The most common reason for a sudden onset of side effects or ineffectiveness is a change in the generic drug manufacturer. Although the active ingredients are relatively consistent, there can be as much as a 15 percent difference in amount, and the fillers that are used may vary and cause side effects. There are a couple of generic manufacturers that tend to cause more side effects. Please ask your pharmacist or your prescriber about their experiences with specific generics.

Will I have ADHD for the rest of my life?

ADHD is a lifelong condition. Treatment and support needs may vary over one's lifetime. Well-managed transitions between key developmental life stages for people with ADHD are important to ensure continuity of adequate care. Many individuals with ADHD stop taking their medications during adolescence and early adulthood, resulting in increased anxieties. Barriers to proper treatment include inadequate ADHD education in primary care,[53] lack of expert services for referral of adults with ADHD,[54] lack of planning, differences in service delivery models

---

[53] C. Brendan Montano and Joel Young, "Discontinuity in the Transition from Pediatric to Adult Health Care for Patients with Attention-Deficit/Hyperactivity Disorder," *Postgraduate Medicine*, 124(5) (2012): 23–32, https://doi.org/10.3810/pgm.2012.09.2591.

[54] David R. Coghill, "Organisation of services for managing ADHD," *Epidemiology and Psychiatric Science*, 26(5) (2016): 453–458, https://doi.org/10.1017/S2045796016000937.

between adult and mental health practices,[55] gaps in communication between child and adult practices,[56] and perceived unhelpful attitudes of some health-care professionals.[57] There is a strong need to ensure clear education of providers and encouragement for children and young adults to continue taking their medication as they transition through different life stages.

SUBSTANCE USE DISORDERS AND STIMULANTS

AADPA guidelines note that substance use disorders will occur in 15 percent of people with ADHD, in contrast to 5.6 percent of the general population.[58]

Treatment for people with both ADHD and substance use disorders should focus on both disorders concurrently, consider their interrelationship, and follow both the guidelines for each separate disorder and the general guidelines about treatment of people with co-occurring disorders. In most cases of concurrent ADHD and substance use disorders, one should begin

---

[55] Tamsin Ford, "Transitional care for young adults with ADHD: transforming potential upheaval into smooth progression," *Epidemiology and Psychiatric Science*, 29 (2020): e87, https:doi.org/10.1017/S2045796019000817.

[56] Charlotte L. Hall, et al., "'Mind the gap'—mapping services for young people with ADHD transitioning from child to adult mental health services," *BMC Psychiatry*, 13 (2013): 186, https://doi.org/10.1186/1471-244X-13-186.

[57] Lauren Matheson, et al., "Adult ADHD patient experiences of impairment, service provision and clinical management in England: a qualitative study," *BMC Health Services Research*, 13 (2013): 184, https://doi.org/10.1186/1472-6963-13-184.

[58] Timothy E. Wilens and Himanshu P. Upadhyaya, "Impact of substance use disorder on ADHD and its treatment," *Journal of Clinical Psychiatry*, 68(8) (2007): e20, https://www.psychiatrist.com/jcp/impact-substance-disorder-adhd-treatment/.

treatment aimed at abstaining from or reducing/stabilizing the use of substances first, since current substance use disorders may complicate diagnosis and treatment of ADHD. However, starting pharmacological or non-pharmacological treatment of ADHD should not be delayed unnecessarily. Pharmacological treatment of ADHD requires careful titration and monitoring of both the beneficial and possible adverse effects. Higher doses of stimulants may be required in people with ADHD with concurrent substance use disorders than in those without substance use disorders to achieve a favorable effect on both the ADHD symptoms and reduction of substance use.

"Tell someone close to you that you're trying a different medication. Sometimes we don't notice changes in ourselves, but they are very clear to someone else. For example, a few days after starting a new medication, my husband pointed out to me that I'd become short-tempered with our children and very focused on the house being immaculately organized. It turns out the dosage was too high; these changes disappeared with a lower dose."

"An unexpected and welcome benefit has been that I have given up drinking every evening as a way to wind down since taking my meds all day long. I feel calmer, more able to focus on my partner and sometimes do some projects in the evening."

CHAPTER 8 PEARLS

1. The first goal is to find the right medication; 90 percent of the time it will be a stimulant (amphetamine or methylphenidate).

2. Then determine the precise dosage; it is not a range.

3. Finally, be sure you are wearing your "focus medicine" all day long, for 12 to 16 hours.

4. You will feel calmer, more able to complete tasks, have more energy, possibly sleep better, and be in a better mood because of proper medication, dosing, and timing of the medicine.

5. Side effects are rare and generally mean you should try either the other stimulant or decrease the dose.

6. Use of alcohol and other substances will likely decrease once you use stimulants correctly.

7. There is no long-term risk of medical disorders or of becoming addicted to ADHD medications.

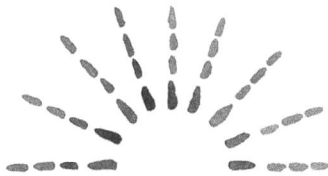

CHAPTER 9

Organizational Strategies: Time Management, Memory, and Clutter

Using a reminder on my phone was a life saver to get into the habit of remembering to take my medication on time. I felt a lot of improvement at first, and now it has evened out, and I feel like every day is full of choices for myself on how I want to spend it without the anxiety and fear that clouded my day before I started on meds. Pills don't build skills, so I've had to learn how to schedule my time better.

Most people with ADHD have executive functioning challenges. These functions include attention control, inhibition, problem solving, and working memory, which requires a fair amount of mental flexibility. You need to

executive functions
The group of complex mental processes and cognitive abilities required for goal-directed behavior.

remember earlier parts of a multistep project, be able to adjust midway through, inhibit distracting stimuli, consider new variables that may appear, and then integrate them into the final product. This translates into difficulties planning, initiating, staying on track, completing tasks, recalling conversations, and keeping track of belongings.

Executive functioning is essential for cognitive, social, and emotional development. So, what happens when a person struggles with planning, monitoring, and executing a project? Some describe it as spinning their wheels or multitasking but not completing a single goal. This is frustrating for those living with people with ADHD and even more devastating to the person who has many unfinished dreams.

One of my favorite quotes from a client is, "When I have a routine, I don't have to have willpower." The irony is that the ADHD brain thrives under a schedule with externally imposed deadlines—an urgent need established by an authority other than oneself to complete a task on time. However, the same ADHD brain does not like doing things in a consistent, robot-like fashion—repeating the same behaviors, in sequence, day after day. Rather, the ADHD brain craves spontaneity and freedom.

This is where you leverage the part of yourself that has learned that doing some things consistently will allow more freedom to be creative or have fun. Sadly, another phrase I've learned from my clients is "revenge bedtime." This refers to feeling that you are owed late-night time to do your own things, because you've been forced to do all the mundane parts of life earlier in the day. This often

> **revenge bedtime**
> Staying up late because you feel you're owed some special alone time to do what you want. Can lead to chronic sleep loss.

applies to parents and working couples who crave time to play video games, surf the internet, or watch favorite shows, not to pursue special hobbies or learn new skills.

A client struggled with addiction in his 20s. He attended AA every day and had a sponsor help him to create a positive routine. He sought treatment for his ADHD and was one of the 10 to 15 percent who don't respond well to stimulants. He decided in his mid-30s to go to law school and was very frustrated that the drugs didn't help. This constraint helped him to be creative. He discovered that if he did the same morning routine every day—ate oatmeal and blueberries, wore one of three pairs of pants and seven T-shirts, and got in a morning run—he could show up at work on time. At work, he created systems to help him meet deadlines. After work each day, he studied with a specific methodology that included printing briefs and highlighting and making special notes that he then brought to class in the evening. He graduated in the top 10 percent of his class and managed to accomplish this *with* systems and *without* stimulants. He also relied on his AA group meetings and his partner for support. This client is unusual, but his story highlights the power of routine, support, and the drive needed to perform well enough to accomplish big goals.

Medication management is fantastic and will greatly improve your quality of life, but just being more focused does not necessarily help with starting important, but often boring, tasks. What helps people with ADHD get started, stay on track, and finish a task?

"I used to spend all my energy setting up my space and establishing new systems. I have so many schedules and special-colored pencils that sadly I used for a week

and then stopped. Now I have a random playlist that I have programmed for the same time every morning that helps me run through my morning chores. The music changes, but the order of my chores stays the same. I'm on autopilot and the new music keeps things interesting and consistent. I haven't forgotten to feed the dog or brush my teeth since I started this method."

EXECUTIVE FUNCTION SUPPORT STRATEGIES

General Considerations

- ☀ Since you can focus on interesting things, make important but boring things more interesting with music, games, or apps.

- ☀ Create accountability by telling someone you are doing the task.

- ☀ Take a step-by-step approach to tasks; rely on visual organizational aids.

- ☀ Use supportive tools like time organizers, computers, or watches with alarms.

- ☀ Prepare visual schedules and review them several times a day. A sturdy, bright, lined notebook works well to create your daily to-do lists.

- ☀ Ask for written directions to supplement verbal instructions whenever possible.

- ☀ Exercise five times a week for 30 minutes; this increases norepinephrine and dopamine and promotes neurogenesis.

☀ Plan and structure transition times and shifts in activities.

☀ Ask for shorter deadlines for part of the assignment from teachers, bosses, parents, and partners.

> **neurogenesis**
> The growth of brain cells.

☀ Expect to be a bumblebee, flitting from one place to another. You are developing a valuable, diverse skill set.

☀ Choose work or an academic area of study that has a lot of variety and sparks passion.

☀ Include time to just "be," so there is balance with the pressure to always "do."

Getting things done doesn't just happen. There is an order to the puzzle of how we manage to get started, stay on track, manage the task, prioritize, and then plan for the next task or event.

Getting Started

☀ Create urgency; make sure there's a deadline and that someone besides you will help keep you accountable.

☀ Just do some part of the task; anything will move you forward.

☀ We procrastinate because we are often afraid of failing at the task; remind yourself that you have done similar tasks and succeeded.

☀ Talk to yourself the way you might to a friend who is struggling.

☀ Ask another person to be a "body double." Set a time when each of you is working on something and schedule a time to check in with each other.

Managing Time

☀ Assess if you struggle with "time blindness." A common expression for people with ADHD's sense of time being "now" and "not now," making planning difficult.

☀ Set timers and alarms before you begin, knowing that you may lose track of time.

☀ Create a "To-Do" List Notebook, breaking down tasks to steps of less than 30 minutes each. Be sure there's only one to-do list, only including things for today, and try to limit your list to five items. If you accomplish more than what is on your list, add the completed task to today's list after completion. Keep your old lists to review when you feel discouraged.

☀ Keep a separate section in your To-Do List Notebook for long-term projects. This is a good place to note things that pop up during the day, so you can stop thinking about them at the moment.

☀ Keep your notebook handy. I suggest a bright color and hardback; it and your phone should be with you all the time.

☀ Break longer assignments into chunks and assign timeframes for completing each chunk.

☀ Prioritize your tasks. If Mom is coming to visit tomorrow, what are the must-do action items?

☀ Use visual calendars to keep track of long-term assignments, due dates, chores, and activities. Alternatively, use life and project management software such as the Franklin Day Planner, Trello, or similar programs.

> **time blindness**
> Difficulty knowing how much time has passed or how long something will take to complete.

☀ Consider using a dry-erase calendar in a central location to track the family's schedule, or an electronic one that syncs with each member's digital calendar.

☀ Whether digital or paper, be sure to include the due date at the top of each assignment.

☀ Short-burst, don't multi-task. Complete one hyper focused activity or task at a time.

☀ Check out the Pomodoro Technique of task completion: Work for a set amount of time—often 20 or 25 minutes—and break for 5 or 10 minutes. The trick is to be firm about returning to work after the break.

☀ Plan for the three parts of a task—setup, work, cleanup—not just the event itself. Build in time for breaks and correcting mistakes.

"When I was a kid, my dad would sit down and go through my homework with me. He'd lay it out on the table and put one little mini candy bar next to each assignment. I got to have one at the start of each piece of homework. It made me happy that he gave me them at the start of each assignment. I wanted to start a new one so I could have the next candy bar. He also left the best ones for the final homework, Snickers and Reese's."

Managing Workspace and Materials

☀ Choose the best space for the project. It might be a noisy coffee shop or a special desk or chair where you only focus on your work.

☀ Consider having separate work areas, with complete sets of supplies, for different activities. If possible, don't combine work and hobbies in one space.

☀ Organize your workspace. Only put things on your desk that you use every week (including fidget toys).

☀ Minimize clutter and make use of drawers and cabinets. "Out of sight" can help a person focus better on the task at hand.

☀ Schedule a weekly time to clean and organize your workspace or have a five-minute music break to tidy things up at the end of each day.

☀ Consider what background music or podcasts help you get things done.

☀ For cooking/baking/any project: Gather all ingredients, bowls, tools, and measuring devices before you start the recipe.

☀ Set up your beverage station so that everything you need is within arm's reach—machine, filter, coffee/tea/water, cups, and any add-ins, like sweetener.

"I used to get so overwhelmed by projects that my husband asked me to do. I felt terrible about myself. Now I tell my sister and neighbor what and when I'm going to do something, and I limit the task to two 30-minute parts. I ask them to check back with me at a specific time to see how I'm doing."

Self-Regulation

※ Recognize that your creative brain and heartfelt purpose will help you generate new ideas and meaningful interactions.

※ Practice nonjudgmental mindfulness; learn to do breathing exercises that help to redirect frustration with your struggles to focus.

※ Practice daily meditation. Even a period of 5 to 10 minutes has been shown to be one of the most effective ways to quiet an anxious mind.

※ Be gentle with your self-talk.

※ Count on regular supportive routines like morning exercise, walking meditation, making a big soup or casserole on Sunday for the week's lunches, breaking for lunch, and scheduling regular times to talk with family and friends. Check your planner and appreciate what you accomplished today and what you plan to do tomorrow.

※ Schedule time to play, and open time for hobbies or other fun activities.

※ For new projects, set a completion date and another to evaluate whether to continue it. It's okay to change direction.

※ If you struggle with impulsive online shopping, try implementing a rule that you can only purchase an item after it has been in your shopping cart for at least 24 hours. This will give you a day to reconsider if you really need this item.

"I can get completely lost in an interesting project. Sometimes I just don't want to stop because I'm afraid that if I stop, I won't come back and finish it. This has resulted in many short nights of sleep and missed engagements. I completely missed my cousin's birthday party because I was so busy working on my motorcycle. I was so embarrassed."

I FEEL STUCK

Remember that your brain is motivated by stimulating, urgent, new, or interesting things. These experiences release dopamine, the "feel good" neurotransmitter. Figure out a way to make a necessary task more exciting or check out what the emotional barrier might be and address that.

When an item on your to-do list has been there for a couple of days and you feel a lot of resistance to doing it, ask yourself what you are feeling about the task. Be curious and write down your response in the next line in your notebook. For example, "I'm scared my email won't be perfect," or "They'll write back, and I'll have even more work to do." Just describing the hard feeling helps release it and can make getting started easier.

Analysis paralysis is real. Sometimes you must open a blank document and write "I don't know how to start" and then continue with whatever stream of consciousness words follow.

Once you have completed an item, let that accomplishment sink in for a moment before moving onto the next item on your to-do list.

Create an immediate reward for completing extra-hard items. This might be listening to a favorite song or eating or drinking something you love while you are doing the task. Consider reserving an extra special treat for only the hardest tasks.

Set the difficult task in motion. For example, if you feel resistance to exercise, begin by putting on your sneakers and then asking yourself if you want to walk, jog, or work out. Sometimes just a bit of momentum will reduce the sense of "stuckness." If you are having trouble cleaning up, invite a friend over later, forcing you to clean up before they arrive. Notice how you feel when you do the important task you don't like. Relief? Associate that good feeling with the accomplishment of the difficult task, to encourage more of the same.

If you can't do the thing for your "today self," consider doing it on behalf of your "tomorrow self." What will the "tomorrow you" feel like if you wake up to a dirty kitchen, or no laundry, or an incomplete assignment? Do something nice for tomorrow you.

Move Around

Movement matters. Get a yoga ball, get up and walk around, use a standing desk, take a 20-minute walk around the building, or go outside. Have phone meetings while walking outside if you don't need your computer or notes. If you are struggling to focus, try walking stairs for 5 or 10 minutes. Stand up and stretch for a short time. All of these can shift energy and support your resilience.

> *"I manage a company and supervise 18 people. My habit was to stay at work until 7 p.m., come home and have dinner with my husband, and then start back up with work duties around 9 and work until 1 a.m. almost every night. I also felt like I deserved to drink a few glasses of wine since I was working*

so hard. Once I started Adderall, and made my mind up to set limits, my work became much more efficient. I was able to delegate to my colleagues, and I told my boss I'd be leaving at 6 p.m. Now I only bring work home once or twice a week. My husband and I actually have 'us' time in the evenings. My weight and blood pressure have also gone way down. I have my life back."

Managing Work

Plan with the end in mind. One strategy is to plan backward: If the big paper is due Friday morning at 9 a.m., then Thursday you spend two hours completing the conclusion, references, and final edits; Wednesday, spend two hours writing the second and third section; Tuesday, spend two hours writing the introduction and first section; Monday, spend two hours completing your research and writing your outline; and over the weekend, you spend three hours doing research.

At school or work, meet with a teacher or supervisor on a regular basis to review work. In these meetings, troubleshoot problems, being sure to agree upon specific outcome measures. Hand in the project or assignment on time, even if it's not perfect. Lower the bar. It's just as important to know when to stop as it is to know how to start. Set firm stop times and leave yourself a note explaining what you worked on last and what needs to be done next.

Seek out a work partner—a friend or family member who is working on something at the same time, whether in the same room or elsewhere. Text them and set up an hour for you both to focus on completing your task of choice. At the end of the time, check in to see how it went and if you want to extend the time or schedule another session.

Group related tasks together: Check emails two or three times a day and block out time to respond; let people know when you check your email; do laundry once a week and clean the laundry area at the same time.

Do Less

Delegate areas of responsibility rather than single jobs, so that you don't have to manage the area. For example, gain agreement that your partner is entirely responsible for taking care of the animals and you'll do the laundry, instead of you each doing part of both jobs. Keep things simple. For example, underwear and T-shirts don't have to be folded when you put them away. Do one thing at a time, at home and work.

> *"Even though the stimulant helped me finish tasks once I had finally started them, it wasn't that helpful in getting started. I had to find ways to motivate myself to do the thing that I had been procrastinating about. I came up with some systems that basically boil down to creating patterns and staying accountable to other people. It also really helps me to have a deadline. I no longer forget to take my meds and my supplements since I started taking them all at the same time, and I fill my pill boxes ahead of time twice a month. It is such a relief to know that I'm taking my meds consistently, and now I've started adding a couple of tasks before I take my meds, like feeding the animals and starting the coffee pot."*

Time- (and Frustration-) Savers

☀ Consider hiring people to do things that have costly consequences if you make mistakes or that you hate to do, such as preparing taxes, small business billing, legal arrangements, house cleaning, and yard work.

☀ Set up regular bills for autopayment.

☀ If you regularly overdraw banking accounts, set up low balance or overdraft alerts.

☀ Create four weekly food shopping lists you can cycle through.

☀ Simplify getting dressed by buying multiple pairs of the same socks, underwear, etc.

☀ Set up a defined place to keep your keys and wallet.

☀ Have a visible clock in every room.

☀ Use electronic tracking devices for important items, like keys, wallet, and your To-Do List Notebook.

☀ Do daily tasks in a set order: get up, use the bathroom, meditate for five minutes, turn on morning music or a podcast, turn on the coffee pot, feed the dog, put away the clean dishes, get dressed, make the bed, eat breakfast, gather things together for the day, brush your teeth, style your hair, and put on makeup.

- Set up not one, but three alarms for leaving the house or starting your workday on time: one to give you a 15-minute warning, another a 5-minute warning, and the last a 2-minute warning.

- Be sure to build in downtime. If those tasks take 40 minutes to complete, then be sure you've given yourself 60 to 80 minutes from when you get out of bed to when you must leave the house or be at your first Zoom meeting.

※ Use smart devices to automate household needs—lighting, thermostat, security, entertainment, vacuums, and more.

※ If you travel often, keep a travel bag with all the essentials—electric cords and plugs, toiletries, sets of underwear, a change of clothes—to be ready to go.

※ Adopt a 20-minute daily cleanup. This works well after dinner. Everyone participates in either cleaning up the kitchen and doing dishes or some other household tasks for just 20 minutes.

- Everyone chooses one to three songs that will be added to a cleanup playlist. I suggest choosing upbeat or edgy tunes, not your or your family's regular favorites.

- Write down chores of 20 minutes or less on poker chips or some other reusable surface in permanent marker and toss them into a bowl. This could include picking up the living room, vacuuming, starting or folding laundry, cleaning the bathroom or kitchen floor, watering the plants, or tidying a bedroom. Be sure to put completed chips in a separate dish to not pull the same chip out the next time. Some people enjoy adding a "Your Choice" and/or a "Do double chores but you choose" chip.

Digital Applications

☀ Some of the best time management digital apps for ADHD (at the time of this writing) include: Clockify, Todoist, Focus@Will, TickTick, Forest, Asana, Priority Matrix, Sunsama, Time Timer, Trello, Amazing Marvin, Habitica, Evernote, Rescue Time, and Remember the Milk. Find one that works for you and use it.

"Before my ADHD was treated, I was buried in sticky notes. I had lots of colors, but I forgot my systems and got overloaded. Since using the To-Do List Notebook system, I'm less anxious because I know everything is in one place. I also love to check things off, and it feels good to look back over the weeks and see how much I've accomplished. My confidence is so much better now that I have a way of tracking what I need to do. I keep the list short and doable. My notebook feels like a friend and not a taskmaster. I even named her Tuti."

Memory

☀ Understand that your working memory is impaired, and the ability to hold new information while working with it—like remembering the name of a restaurant while you are looking for a pen to jot down the restaurant's name—is limited. "Out of sight, out of mind" makes remembering to retrieve the jacket you brought to school challenging.

☀ Keep a calendar of important dates—birthdays, anniversaries—so that your family and friends don't assume you just don't care.

☀ Snap bracelets can be helpful reminders. Try keeping a few of them in the kitchen, bedroom, and office. Put one on when you must remember to do something in the next hour or two, like take out the garbage or let the dog back in.

☀ Sticky notes are good for short-term reminders. Put one on the corner of your laptop to remind you to add a task to your To-Do List Notebook. Don't use it as your actual task reminder. Keep the list in only one place—your To-Do List Notebook—not on your phone, the fridge, desk, etc.

☀ Some people prefer a work notebook and a home notebook, while others use the front for home and back for work, eventually meeting in the middle, and the notebook goes everywhere you go.

☀ Ask your friends and family to gently remind you of events a day and again two hours in advance.

☀ Some people appreciate being told an event starts 30 minutes before it actually starts. This way they can relax when they think they are late and actually arrive a few minutes early. If this is you, it can reinforce the good feeling of arriving on time.

☀ Make the content of what you just studied, read, or had a meeting about into a story, act it out, or create a song or drawing to help your brain remember it. Even better, teach the content to someone else.

Sleep

Sleep is the foundation of all mental health. Getting better sleep improves test scores and overall functioning and performance.[59] Practice good sleep hygiene:

☀ Shut down all electronics and blue light devices one hour before bed.

- If you must use your device in that hour, adjust your settings to dim the light and set it to a warm color (such as amber) rather than a brighter one (blue). *This is truly for exceptions only.*

☀ Darken the room in which you sleep and lower the temperature.

☀ Stop drinking liquids two hours before bed; stop caffeine intake by 2 p.m.

☀ Listen to relaxing shows or music before sleep.

☀ Check with your care provider when considering if 240 to 480 mg of magnesium glycinate, 1 to 1.5 mg melatonin ER, or lemon balm is a helpful supplement that fits well with your other meds or supplements.

☀ Go to bed and wake up at consistent times, even on the weekend.

☀ Avoid conflicts before bed. Don't discuss hard topics while in bed.

☀ Do all you can to invite your brain to associate your bed only with sleep, snuggling, and sex.

---

[59] David L. Chandler, "Study: Better sleep habits lead to better college grades," *MIT News* (2019), https://news.mit.edu/2019/better-sleep-better-grades-1001.

※ Get cozy, good smelling, soft or firm pillows, weighted blankets, comfy sheets, and the right (or no) sleepwear.

※ Adopt what makes you feel safe and relaxed.

※ Honor your natural circadian rhythm (are you an early bird or a night owl?) and set your sleep schedule accordingly.

※ If you can, leave your phone in another room and use one or more alarms to wake up, with the final, loudest one being set on your phone.

※ Keep a stack of sticky notes and a pen next to your bed. If you have a thought about something you need to do, jot it down and then add it to your To-Do List Notebook in the morning.

※ Prepare for morning by setting out your clothes and packing your lunch the night before.

※ Use smart lightbulbs that gradually dim at night and brighten in the morning.

※ If you wake up in the night, practice meditation or get out of bed and read. Don't get on your phone and don't remain in bed.

Clutter and Organization

There are many suggestions for how to declutter and organize your living space. Check out Marie Kondo, a household decluttering celebrity, and the theory of minimalism. Find a system that works for you until you get bored with it and then change it.

Expect to have some degree of clutter, but how much is too much for you?

- ☀ If you haven't used something that has been out for 24 hours, put it back in its place. If it doesn't have a place, create one or get rid of it.
- ☀ Set up and use well-placed containers such as laundry baskets, shoe racks, coat racks, toy chests, dirty dishes bins, and recycling and trash bins in multiple rooms.
- ☀ Use a basket at the top and bottom of stairs for things that need to be transported between floors.

Work to clear clutter in your home and workspace, and create a place for each of your belongings. This will also help clear your brain to enable it to focus on important goals.

Making all your spaces work with and for you can be calming and aid in getting your day or work started. Consider room-specific organization strategies:

- ☀ In the bathroom, install several hooks for towels and organize toiletries in baskets. Maintain a refill shelf stocked with toilet paper, toothpaste, soap, shampoo, and razors.
- ☀ In the kitchen, make sure that everything has a logical place. Shelve baking pans together, put pots together, place mugs near the coffee pot, and so forth.
- ☀ In your bedroom closet, label bins for accessories on a shelf, sort shirts into short and long sleeves, and group pants into casual, jeans, and dress. Consider collapsable shirt or pant racks as well.

☀ Create zones in your home entryway. Use hooks for backpacks and coats, shelves or racks for shoes, and a special place for keys.

☀ Place your sports gear all in one place, in labeled bins: all of the ski clothes, helmets, and goggles in one; biking repair kits, extra tubes, tools, water bottle, and helmet in another.

"Before treatment, I didn't understand the importance of creating systems to keep my spaces tidy. After treatment, I now know that for me, everything must have a place, and once it does, it is much easier to put things away, which in turn makes it a lot easier to keep my spaces tidy."

"This is my own story. I hate unloading the dishwasher. I don't mind loading it, but unloading it is not my thing. Every time I go to open the door, I have to convince myself that just putting the clean plates on the counter above the plate drawer is easy. Then I look at the rack and think, the bowls aren't too bad. Then there's a few random things like the cheese grater. Now I only have the utensil basket, ugh. Okay, I'll take it out and put it on the counter over the silverware drawer. I gingerly pull out the top rack. The mugs are fairly easy too, and the glasses follow. I don't like dealing with plastic containers and lids; they are still wet. I'll just put them on top of my gas stove so they can dry and deal with them later. Now I only have a few more items like little bowls. Those aren't too hard. Sometimes I close the door, but then I feel bad because it's closed without the silverware basket being returned. Darn. Okay, I'll put away the silverware. The knives are the easiest; next come the spoons and finally the forks which I find confusing because the dinner and salad size are so similar.

This entire process might take me 5 or 10 minutes, but it feels like a huge accomplishment, and just putting that first plate away starts the cascade, one step at a time."

PROJECT EXAMPLE: CLEANING OUT YOUR CLOSET

Getting Started

☀ Tell two people you are going to clean out your closet this week.

☀ Get three boxes and label them Toss, Give Away, and Sort.

☀ Choose one small part of the closet to clean out, setting a timer for 20 minutes.

☀ Start with the thing you are most interested in, rather than what you should do.

☀ Choose harder projects when your brain is most alert, such as after exercising.

Maintaining Momentum

☀ Throw out the trash, put the first giveaway box in the car, and get another one.

☀ Set a timer for 20 minutes, sit down, and begin processing the "Sort" box. Making it a 20-minute assignment helps the task be more manageable.

☀ Push to keep going, even if it's just doing one tiny thing such as putting one item from the box into its proper place.

☀ Tell a friend if you want to give up or are feeling overwhelmed.

☀ Rather than forcing yourself to "do," invite yourself to be curious about being done.

☀ Celebrate the thing you did right or are challenged to do better, rather than fixating on what went wrong.

CHAPTER 9 PEARLS

1. Employ a routine so you don't have to muster as much willpower.

2. Make things interesting by using music, apps, or games.

3. Create urgency; tell someone you are going to complete a task by a specific time.

4. Use a single, lined To-Do List Notebook as the only place you write down tasks.

5. Set up separate spaces for school or work and play in your home.

6. Break tasks down into 20- to 30-minute subtasks.

7. Use timers and alarms.

8. Create a big family calendar in a central location.

9. Meet with your teacher, boss, and partner to discuss plans regularly.

10. Write it down.

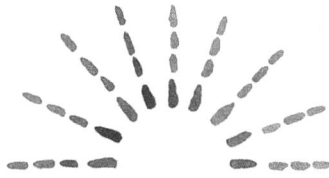

CHAPTER 10

Women and ADHD, with a Focus on Workplace Considerations

My mother, my boss, even my husband said I couldn't possibly have ADHD because I'm "a smart girl" and I have a master's degree and am not hyper. I was so tired of trying extra hard, staying up late, always struggling with details, and waiting until the last minute to get my focus in gear. My counselor noticed that the three different antidepressants I'd tried didn't seem to help my mood and that I was always struggling with time management and deadlines. I was exhausted all the time. Once I started with my ADHD Nurse Practitioner, things started to fall into place. She told me that even though I'm five foot one, 110 pounds, and female, I might still need a higher dose of stimulant. That's what happened. I now take Vyvanse twice a day since it wears off after six hours, and my mother, boss, and husband have all

*commented that I'm so much more productive and happier.
I stopped my Lexapro prescription from my other provider,
and I have time after work to do things with my husband and
not just watch TV. I only wish I'd known this 20 years ago.*

DIFFERENCES FOR GIRLS AND WOMEN

Women's rates of ADHD in adulthood are nearly the same as men. Unfortunately, they are far more likely to be diagnosed as adults than men, who are more than twice as likely to be diagnosed as children. The misconception that girls who are smart and dreamy or anxious and depressed don't have ADHD has resulted in more women either going undiagnosed or only discovering late into adulthood that they have been living with ADHD.

The misperception we discussed earlier—that ADHD describes a hyperactive person who can't attend—often means these women, their medical providers, and their therapists do not understand that the root cause of many of their struggles are difficulties attending to important details, a hyperactive and at times impulsive brain, and a significant amount of mood dys-regulation or RSD. For those diagnosed later in life, sometimes in their 50s, 60s, or 70s, there is a tremendous sense of loss.

Common comments that clients have shared include: "If I'd only known earlier." "Why didn't anyone recognize this?" "What would my life have been like if I'd been treated as a child, or in college, or even when I first started my family?" Hopefully in the future we will come to recognize ADHD earlier in all children.

Boys tend to take their frustrations out on others—the classic disruptive boy in the classroom or playground many of us picture when we think of a child with ADHD. On the other hand, girls tend to internalize their problems and are more prone to anxiety, depression, and rumination. They may not be physically hyperactive, but their minds are racing much of the time. They feel ashamed about feeling different and overwhelmed, become very adept at hiding their feelings, and sometimes become "people-pleasers."

Cultural norms also contribute to the necessity for women to juggle their own needs, the needs of their family, and work or school responsibilities. Men with ADHD are more likely to be able to just get by or hyperfocus on their jobs and not have to also take on most of the care of the home and children. Women often feel like they are imposters and tend to be self-critical when comparing themselves to their peers. The degree of self-judgment and doubt about their capability can become overwhelming and lead to further anxiety and depression.

As a result of gender norms, girls and women are more likely to compensate by hyperfocusing on the thing they think their parent, teacher, or boss wants and then be exhausted and struggle to take care of daily tasks for the remainder of their day. Sometimes this behavior results in parents, teachers, bosses, and even medical professionals not recognizing the person's ADHD, telling her there is nothing wrong with her and she should just try harder.

Additionally, girls and women are also impacted by hormonal differences. Hormone fluctuations that occur in girls and women in premenstrual cycles, pregnancy, perimenopause, and menopause all contribute to an increase in ADHD symptoms, making diagnosis of the root cause, ADHD, often seem more consistent with anxiety or depression. Estrogen improves cognition, and when it wanes, struggles with attention, memory, and mood can inhibit the ability to concentrate. Estrogen modulates executive functions, attention, verbal memory, sleep, concentration, motivation, and neurotransmitter activity. Put simply, as estrogen decreases, ADHD symptoms increase. Often a woman's internal experience and degree of impairment or level of anxiety lead to a "fake it until you make it" coping strategy, which is extremely taxing and, over time, debilitating.

> *"Before I got into college and eventually went to medical school, I used to skip English and history class and go to the park and read my books and underline them and reread them. I couldn't learn by listening to my teachers when it came to 'talking' classes. I was good at math and science when we were 'doing' things, but I just spaced out in classes where the teacher just lectured. I had very few friends because it took me three times as long to do my homework, because I was so distracted and anxious all the time. It wasn't until I got diagnosed in medical school that I finally got some help. I never want anyone else to have to go through what I did."*

When a girl can't concentrate socially and academically, she is more likely to be bullied, left out of groups, and considered lazy or stupid. Consequently, she will become anxious and often eventually depressed. The amount of effort it takes to do basic tasks of everyday living and get through school, and eventually work, is overwhelming and can lead to self-medicating with alcohol, cannabis, or addicting behaviors like online shopping or gambling.

Even more alarming, the rates of self-harm, unplanned pregnancy, and suicide are much higher in girls with ADHD.

Stephen Hinshaw, PhD, has conducted research on girls and women with ADHD since 1997. He noted that by age 20, one out of four girls with ADHD have made a serious attempt on their own life. Over half are engaged in self-harm behaviors, such as cutting and burning themselves.[60,61]

Girls and women with ADHD tend to be more socially isolated. They are less likely to initiate friendships and have fewer meaningful relationships than their peers, in part because they have trouble prioritizing and managing their schedules. Because of their rejection sensitivity, they are more likely to believe that they have failed or have said or done the wrong thing. This is true even when their friends and family reassure them that they are not angry or upset with them. Their self-judgment is very overdeveloped, undermining and often interfering with their ability to enjoy and appreciate the extent to which their loved ones value and love them. This may be the most heartbreaking aspect of ADHD. These intuitive, creative, heartfelt women are excessively focused on their perceived failures and are too often unable to internalize how loved and appreciated they are. Unfortunately, some women will deal with over-stimulation by self-medicating and isolating themselves from others.

Physical complaints are more common in women with ADHD than men with ADHD. These include headaches, migraines, stomachaches, nausea, or fibromyalgia. Insomnia is much more likely in women with ADHD than women without ADHD. All of

---

[60] Rodrigo Pérez Ortega, "Under-diagnosed and under-treated, girls with ADHD face distinct risks," *Knowable Magazine* (2020), https://knowablemagazine.org/article/mind/2020/adhd-in-girls-and-women.

[61] Stephen Hinshaw, PhD., "Girls and Women with ADHD," *ADDitude* Magazine (2018), https://www.youtube.com/watch?v=5y6W9C4rJXw.

this makes concentration and mood regulation more difficult. There can also be sensory issues, like sensitivity to sound, chewing, light changes, or strong odors.

As a result of untreated ADHD, the likelihood of comorbid conditions—anxiety, depression, eating disorders, and more—in women with ADHD increases greatly. They may also be more likely to participate in risky behaviors like speeding, hypersexuality, compulsive shopping, addictions, and bulimia. Research in recent years has shown that women with ADHD are twice as likely as men with ADHD and the general population to die of accidental death.[62] Life expectancy may be reduced by as much as 13 years, but according to leading ADHD expert Russel Barkley, PhD, this can be mitigated if treated and if lifestyle adjustments are made.[63]

TREATMENT CONSIDERATIONS

The good news is that there is help. The best place to start is to learn more about ADHD in general and how it impacts women specifically. When you are evaluated, be sure that your provider is looking at your biochemistry and genetics. Have them check whether you have the MTHFR gene deficiency and any micronutrient deficiencies uncovered by laboratory analyses. Let those close to you know that you are living with ADHD, which can make it harder for you to concentrate and regulate your moods.

---

[62] Søren Dalsgaard, et al., "Mortality in children, adolescents, and adults with attention deficit hyperactivity disorder: a nationwide cohort study," *The Lancet*, 385 (9983) (2015): 2190–2196, https:doi.org/10.1016/S0140-6736(14)61684-6.

[63] Barkley, "How ADHD Affects Life Expectancy."

Sharing with your family and friends will make learning to live with ADHD much easier.

Once you've improved your diet to include more vegetables and lean protein and are taking any supplements that were recommended based on testing and not guessing, then it is time for the proper and precise use of medications. Refer to the chapter on medication for more exact guidance, but remember there are only two medications: amphetamines, the most common brand name being Adderall, and methylphenidate, brand name Ritalin. Amphetamines often work best. If they don't work, or if they cause anxiety or irritability, change with a provider's oversight to methylphenidate. The dosage is incredibly important. Again, think of the eyeglass analogy. You want the perfect prescription to see with clear vision, and you'll need to wear them whenever you need to focus—all day, every day.

Another word about medication: The difference between taking 7.5 mg, 10 mg, and 12.5 mg can be the difference between "feeling like yourself, just focused" and feeling like you are always struggling with distraction or experiencing additional anxiety. Any side effect with these medications is generally either because you are taking the wrong one of the two options or your dosage is too high. If you find yourself having more symptoms as the medication wears off, then take another similar dose, i.e., put your glasses back on, please.

The fact that you are male or female, young or old, skinny or heavy does not affect your dosage. You must find the right one for you. For some people, that is a mere 5 mg a day; for others, it might be as much as 90 mg or two long-acting preparations. If your blood pressure is stable and you are not experiencing any side effects, then continue to increase your dose by 2.5 mg of short-acting medication per dose until you find the perfect amount. When you "fall off the mountain" and have a side effect, you will recognize that yesterday's dose was the precise dosage you need. The Federal Drug Administration recommends a maximum of 60 mg per day. My clinical experience, and many others', has shown that to cover a 12- to 16-hour day, this dosage is inadequate for 30–40 percent of our clients.

> "For so many years I relied on baseline anxiety and my smarts. I could always figure things out; maybe I'd be a little late, but my contributions were valued. When I hit menopause, I felt like my brain had sludge in it. Things were heavy, confusing, and I got so weepy and irritable, it was awful. My provider suggested I start on hormones, and good heavens, what a difference. Not only do I have some sex drive, but I'm sleeping better and have stopped losing and forgetting things, well at least most of the time. I wish I'd done this in my 50s and did not wait until I was 60. I lost so much self-confidence, and it nearly cost me my job and my relationship. I wish people knew about the importance of getting on HRT and stimulants sooner."

THE IMPACT OF HORMONES: PMS AND MENOPAUSE

Understanding that low estrogen levels impact the ability to concentrate and to regulate mood fluctuations can help clinicians and women living with ADHD recognize that they may need to adjust their dosage of medication during the parts of their menstrual cycle when their estrogen is dipping. Increasing the dose by 20 to 50 percent during these periods may help alleviate the symptoms. Girls and women may benefit from using birth control pills to regulate their menstrual cycles to avoid the monthly decline in estrogen.

Bioidentical hormone replacement therapy for women during and after menopause is a recently understood tool in treating mature women with ADHD. Many providers are unaware of the research supporting the importance of most women using hormones pre-, during, and post-menopause. Most women will spend 30 years or more with estrogen defi-ciency, which causes the common symptoms of drying skin, weaker bones, and hot flashes. In addition, low estrogen levels are also responsible for increases in irritability and a drop in libido, concentration, energy, and sleep quality. Women who do not use hormone replacement therapy, according to Dr. Ann Hathaway, experience a 30 percent increase in the incidence of dementia.[64] Many women who've managed their ADHD with-out stimulant medications most of their life find that they suf-fer from increasing brain fog and memory loss once they enter menopause.

Get a consultation with a skilled provider who specializes in working with hormones. Recent research even supports women with a history of certain kinds of breast cancer being possible candidates for HRT.[65] (The Women's Health Initiative study

---

[64] Ann Hathaway, MD, "Women, Estrogen, Cognition and Alzheimer's Disease," Townsend Letter (June 2012), https://annhathawaymd.com/wp-content/uploads/2012/01/annhathawaymd-topwnsend.pdf.
[65] Diana Schlamadiner, "What Research Says About HRT and Breast Cancer Risk," Breast Cancer Research Foundation (2024), https://www.bcrf.org/about-breast-cancer/hrt-breast-cancer-risk/.

(1991 to 2005) made several claims regarding the risk of cancer due to HRT that have since been refuted.[66])

To summarize ADHD care for women:

1. Educate yourself about ADHD.

2. Find a provider who will prescribe stimulant medications accurately; you may have to educate them based on your own learning.

3. Consult with a health-care practitioner who is familiar with hormone replacement.

4. Consider working with a coach or therapist who understands ADHD to support executive functioning growth.

You may need to go online and find someone outside of your immediate community who is experienced. Reduce isolation and loneliness by joining online support groups. Find your tribe. One word of caution: Be careful about how you talk with friends and family about being treated for ADHD. It remains largely misunderstood, and most of the public and many professionals are uninformed about the extraordinary benefits of using stimulant medications properly. Even more notable, they are not aware of the extent of the life-altering experiences that people living with ADHD experience when their medication boosts their neurotransmitters to a level that supports dramatic improvements in attention and mood. Talk about improving

---

[66] Angelo Cagnacci and Martina Venier, "The Controversial History of Hormone Replacement Therapy," *Medicina*, 55(9) (2019): 602, https:doi.org/10.3390/medicina55090602.

your concentration, mood, and energy, and consider carefully when to use the term "ADHD."

Work Considerations

Remember that your ADHD brain will be drawn to interesting tasks. You will want to choose work that keeps you challenged and probably not sitting at a desk all day. Although routine may help you not have to rely on willpower, you will want to work somewhere that is dynamic, requires you to have a varied approach, and encourages you to move your body during the day. Find a way to incorporate a solid morning and evening routine that supports creative expression during the day. When you can count on yourself to get the required self-care completed at both ends of the day, there is less anxiety and more mental space to have increased creative time during the day.

Consider how you tend to accomplish most tasks. Most people will say when it becomes urgent and there's a clear deadline. People with ADHD often excel in environments where someone else holds them accountable and there are clear consequences for not meeting deadlines. Many professions meet this description, including nursing, teaching, education, accounting, trades, chef, engineering, journalism, event planning, and emergency medicine.

If you are employed, speak with your employer about your ADHD diagnosis and let them know that there are several things that will help you be a better employee. Having weekly check-ins with clear expectations and definitions of your job responsibilities and their deadlines will help keep the guesswork out of your duties. You may find that it is valuable to have your manager break your job down into smaller actions. You may learn better by shadowing another employee rather than listening to or reading about what you are expected to accomplish.

Confirm that your boss wants you to ask clarifying questions, and that you benefit from immediate constructive feedback. Remember that your RSD might get triggered and employ your coping mechanisms to address this early on.

I suggest holding off on sharing your diagnosis until you've been offered the position. Unfortunately, there are still too many negative stereotypes and a lack of knowledge that might support discrimination during the hiring process.

Problems with attention and impulsivity can lead to serious difficulties when needing to concentrate on important repetitive, uninteresting tasks. This can lead to errors, reprimands, and, unfortunately, job loss. The Attention Deficit Disorder Association newsletter reported in its July 2023 edition that one out of three people with ADHD are jobless at any one time.[67]

In this same article, the risks for employees with untreated ADHD are shocking:

☀ **Loss of household income:** People living with ADHD report an annual average loss of household income of $8,900 to $15,400.[68]

---

[67] ADDA Editorial Team, "Impact of ADHD at Work," ADDA.org (2023), https://add.org/impact-of-adhd-at-work/#:~:text=ADHD%20at%20 work%20results%20in,also%20has%20larger%20socioeconomic%20 impacts.

[68] Jalpa A. Doshi, et al., "Economic Impact of Childhood and Adult Attention-Deficit/Hyperactivity Disorder in the United States," *Journal of the American Academy of Child and Adolescent Psychiatry*, 51(10) (2012): 990–1002, https://doi.org/10.1016/j.jaac.2012.07.008.

☀ **Poor productivity:** Adults with untreated ADHD lose an average of 22 days of productivity per year.[69]

☀ **Loss of employment:** Employees with ADHD are 30 percent more likely to have chronic employment issues, 60 percent more likely to be fired from a job, and three times more likely to quit a job impulsively.[70]

☀ **Stress-induced illness:** Another study on the incidence of ADHD reported that at least 24 percent of employees on long-term sick leave due to stress-related illness met the criteria for ADHD.[71]

☀ **Stigma:** Social rejection by peers, minimizing ADHD symptoms, name-calling, lost promotions, bullying, and job termination are only a few examples reported in a 2014–2015 survey by ADDA's Workplace Committee.[72] As a result, ADHDers may experience intense stress as they struggle with shame and guilt, as well as having to work much harder to make up for their productivity challenges.[73]

---

[69] Michael F. Hilton, et al., "The Association Between Mental Disorders and Productivity in Treated and Untreated Employees," *Journal of Occupational and Environmental Medicine*, 51(9) (2009): 996–1003, https://doi.org/10.1097/JOM.0b013e3181b2ea30.

[70] Russell A. Barkley, Kevin R. Murphy, and Mariellen Fischer, *ADHD in Adults: What the Science Says* (Guilford Press, 2010), 279.

[71] Gunilla Brattberg, "PTSD and ADHD: Underlying factors in many cases of burnout," *Stress and Health*, 22 (2006): 305–313, https://doi.org/10.1002/smi.1112.

[72] Linda Walker, "Should You Disclose Your ADHD at Work? Survey Says …" ADDA.org (2016), https://adhdatwork.add.org/should-you-disclose-your-adhd-at-work-survey-says/.

[73] Joseph Biederman and Stephen V. Faraone, "The effects of attention-deficit/hyperactivity disorder on employment and household income," *Medscape General Medicine*, 8(3) (2006): 12, https://pubmed.ncbi.nlm.nih.gov/17406154/.

> **Americans with Disabilities Act (ADA)**
> US law prohibiting discrimination based on disability; also requires employers to provide reasonable accommodations for employees with disabilities.

The most important legal protection for workers with ADHD is the Americans with Disability Act (ADA) of 1990 (amended and expanded in 2008). The ADA is essentially a civil rights law prohibiting discrimination against individuals with "a physical or mental impairment that substantially limits one or more major life activities of such individual."[74] Women are particularly vulnerable to being discriminated against in the workforce. Their need to prioritize their children, the ongoing existence of the glass ceiling, underrepresentation of women leaders, and a preponderance for male-to-female sexual harassment makes the stakes considerably higher.

Another key resource for employers and employees is the Job Accommodation Network (JAN), which offers some very specific recommendations:[75]

Accommodating Employees with Attention Deficit Hyperactivity Disorder (ADHD)

General accommodation for individuals with ADHD addresses the common tendency to be perfectionistic and have trouble with boundary setting. They give the impression that they can handle

---

[74] U.S. Department of Justice, Civil Rights Division, "Introduction to the Americans with Disabilities Act," ADA.gov, accessed July 2025, https://www.ada.gov/topics/intro-to-ada/.

[75] Job Accommodation Network, JAN.org, accessed July 15, 2025, https://askjan.org/.

a heavier workload because of their tendency to overwork and desire to assure their boss that they are competent and willing to work overtime.

General accommodations include:

☀ Identify and focus on strengths; de-emphasize weaknesses.

☀ Emphasize creativity.

☀ Notice when the individual is overworked: not taking vacations, staying at work late frequently, not eating lunch.

☀ Provide an ADHD coach to help improve productivity and maintain a healthy work-life balance.

I recommend JAN's "Accommodation Solutions: Executive Functioning Deficits," detailing accommodations for individuals with limitations related to executive functioning, including ADHD. Not all people with ADHD will need accommodation to perform their jobs, and some may only need a few accommodations. Employers should ask the following questions of employees with ADHD who request accommodation.

Questions to Consider for the Employer:

1. What limitation affects what task, and how does it decrease their performance?

2. What accommodation would address the limitation, and is it being used?

3. How often should the employee and employer meet to evaluate the effectiveness of the accommodation?

4. Do staff and supervisors need any training regarding accommodations?

Visit JAN's website for a comprehensive list.

Examples of Accommodations

Hyperactivity/Impulsivity support

- ☀ Establish regular breaks for movement.
- ☀ Consider a work-from-home arrangement.
- ☀ Suggest a job coach or mentor.
- ☀ Provide information about the Employee Assistance Program (EAP).

Focus/concentration support

- ☀ Create a quiet workspace.
- ☀ Assure regular work breaks.
- ☀ Provide noise cancellation or white noise devices.
- ☀ Optimize focus on interesting tasks and delegate boring tasks, if possible.

Time management

- ☀ Meet regularly: weekly, biweekly, or monthly.
- ☀ Review the employee's to-do list and accomplishments in the meeting.
- ☀ Help the employee prioritize work.
- ☀ Provide timers and calendars as appropriate.

Even with ADA support in the workplace, the employee must also contribute to their own success. See Chapter 9 to find healthy routines that support your success.

While there is a tendency to become overly aware of problems with attention and impulsive behaviors, it is important to note the advantages of living with an interest-based brain. The Journal of Attention Disorders reported in a 2020 study: "We did not observe differences . . . in intrinsic motivation during idea generation between groups, but adults with ADHD generated more original ideas when competing for a bonus."[76]

Focus on the strengths you bring. You were hired because you had the skills and knowledge to do the job. You may find that you are the team member who comes up with new strategies, is able to think outside of the box, and has an uncanny sense of what needs to be addressed in different and often successful ways.

CHAPTER 10 PEARLS

1. Women have nearly the same incidence of ADHD as men but are underdiagnosed.
2. Women are often treated for depression and anxiety, and their ADHD is entirely missed.
3. The risk of self-harm is as high as 25 percent in girls and women under age 20 with ADHD.

---

[76] Nathalie Boot, Barbara Nevicka, and Matthijs Baas, "Creativity in ADHD: Goal-Directed Motivation and Domain Specificity," *Journal of Attention Disorders*, 24(13) (2017): 1857–1866, https://doi.org/10.1177/1087054717727352.

4. A drop in estrogen can lessen a woman's ability to concentrate, requiring an increase in stimulant dosage before menstruation and during menopause.

5. Access the Job Accommodation Network resources for workplace accommodation suggestions.

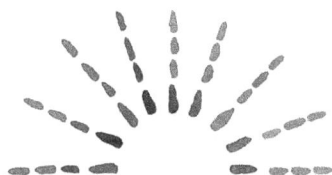

CHAPTER 11

Parenting Children with ADHD

I didn't realize that I had ADHD until after I had my child assessed. When the doctor started listing the common symptoms, I realized that I'd struggled with similar issues and wondered if I should get evaluated too. Once I did, I felt like I was finally wearing glasses after living in a blur all my life. I wish someone had recognized this earlier; even though I was smart, I was working twice as hard as I needed to. I feel like a fog has been lifted.

One of the most common experiences I have as a clinician is acknowledging how hard it is to be diagnosed later in life. "Why didn't my parents recognize this was a problem?" Unfortunately, mostly the answer is because their parents didn't recognize their own ADHD, and the ability to diagnose and treat ADHD remains very limited. The best thing you can do to help your child with ADHD is to investigate whether you, too, have ADHD. Just like the airline safety video says, put on your own oxygen mask before helping your child. Take the online ASRS assessment, and if it's positive, find a provider who will begin a trial of stimulant medication.

A number of books and articles are available on parenting children with ADHD. Here are some basic concepts and guidance that have worked for my clients' families.

TOP NINE PEARLS FOR PARENTING A CHILD WITH ADHD

Over my years of raising children, I have personally failed at most of these. Trial and error, learning what works well for my clients, and studying the experts have demonstrated that these insights and practices are very effective:

1. ADHD is a genetic variation on how brains work. There are strengths—e.g., creativity and heartfulness—in addition to the challenges—e.g., difficulties with concentration and being highly sensitive to criticism. Educate yourself with videos and reading.

2. Get yourself and/or your child's other parent evaluated before seeking treatment for your child.

3. Have your child assessed early and use medications from the beginning.

4. Broccoli, love, and exercise matter. Focus on diet, affection, and movement daily.

5. Routine is paramount. *"When I have a routine, I don't have to have willpower."* Set up your home and your child's schedule for simple success.

6. Support emotional regulation and practice calming techniques together.

7. Teach skills by modeling and giving positive feedback.

8. Access available support—family, friends, and professionals.

9. Take care of yourself. Do not exhaust yourself or overprioritize your child.

EDUCATION

We covered what ADHD is and isn't in Chapter 2. Not everyone presents as "Tigger," all bouncy and energetic. Sometimes the smart but tired and distracted child has attention issues. Often the kid who seems "overly sensitive" and gets waylaid by a friend's remarks has ADHD. Medications are extremely effective 75 percent of the time and are the treatment that experts recommend first, not after everything else has failed.[77] In my clinical experience, with careful titration and additional support of the client's micronutrients, I have seen closer to 90 percent efficacy.

Once you start learning about the extraordinary capacity that you and your child will have when the proper support is put into place, you will begin to dream about living a more mutually successful and happy life. There is no advantage to delaying treatment, and fortunately the difference between applying only the broccoli, love, and exercise approach and adding the precise use of stimulants is life changing.

"I was so focused on getting my son treated that I completely overlooked my own ADHD. The problem was that I was so

[77] Claire Advokat and Mindy Scheithauer, "Attention-Deficit hyperactivity disorder (ADHD) stimulant medications as cognitive enhancers," *Frontiers in Neuroscience*, 7 (2013): 82, https://doi.org/10.3389/fnins.2013.00082.

disorganized that I couldn't help him consistently take the medicine and supplements, never mind building a regular morning and nighttime schedule with him. I feel so bad that I wasted two years of struggling to keep things organized before I finally started taking Ritalin myself."

TREAT YOURSELF FIRST

Even if you can't find an ADHD specialist for yourself or your partner right away, go on a hyperfocused learning jag to gain a solid understanding of what ADHD is all about. Most of us are undereducated or misinformed, as I was when I opened my practice in 2013. Start asking around for local providers who treat ADHD. Ask your pharmacist who they know in your area. Check the national provider list on the add.org website and your local Children and Adults with ADHD (CHADD) chapter for recommendations.

You must wear your "glasses" all day long if you want to stay focused. Use your medications, and be sure to take them all day, every day, and your life will undergo dramatic improvement. If things don't go perfectly with Adderall, try Ritalin. Work through your provider, start at a very low dose, and gradually increase until you find your perfect individualized prescription. Once you've found your precise amount, then add an extended-release medication. You may need a third booster dose in the late afternoon to keep you focused through your child's bedtime.

CHILD EVALUATION AND TREATMENT

Find a skilled provider for your child. Increasingly, many pediatricians are well-versed in treating kids with ADHD, whereas others prefer to refer to a specialist or may require extra testing. Sometimes the psychologists who do the diagnoses can offer a good referral. There are ADHD counselors and coaches who may know the names of qualified providers in town. Additionally, as noted, you can also check with your local pharmacy.

Prepare to put systems in place that will support a detailed and well-documented trial of medications. You will want to be completely sure of what your child's response is and absolutely *do not* use it "as needed." Your goal is to help your child to attend better from morning until night. This will impact their ability to complete tasks in school and at home, which in turn will improve their mood, sense of self, and provide them the confidence to tackle other areas that interest them.

BROCCOLI, LOVE, AND EXERCISE

Diet

In his excellent book, *Finally Focused*, Dr. James Greenblatt recommends starting with an anti-inflammation diet.[78]

He clearly outlines, in order of priority, his recommendations for the treatment of ADHD, starting with diet.

- ☀ Stop eating gluten, sugar, and sometimes dairy.
- ☀ Avoid all processed foods, which are largely lacking in vitamins and minerals and can worsen inattention, hyperactivity, and mood disorders.

---

[78] James Greenblatt, *Finally Focused: The Breakthrough Natural Treatment Plan for ADHD that Restores Attention, Minimizes Hyperactivity, and Helps Eliminate Drug Side Effects* (Harmony Press, 2017).

☀ Do not use or consume foods with corn syrup, white rice, artificial coloring and additives, sodium benzoate, or aspartame.

☀ Stick to whole foods, including fresh organic meats, fruits, vegetables, whole grains, nuts, and seeds.

☀ Be sure to eat enough protein.

Greenblatt recommends testing and not guessing; namely, getting lab work results. Basic supplements to address imbalances could include magnesium glycinate or citrate, zinc, vitamin D3 with K2, vitamin B complex, and omega-3s. In addition, there may be a need for iron, probiotics, amino acids, and plant phenols (like green tea, pine bark, and blueberry extract). Remember my client's story in Chapter 7 about scoring the bullseye on all her labs as a result of eating no processed foods, having daily greens, and enjoying a serving of homemade berry pie?

Love

This cannot be overemphasized. We all long to be accepted and seen for who we are. Children crave acknowledgment from their peers and authority figures, but first and foremost they want to know they are loved and valued by their family. The surest way of connecting deeply with your child is to do what they are doing with them. Get down on the floor and play, go outside, play games, read stories, cook together, and do homework with them. Have them participate in what you are doing; model, teach and support them to do some aspects of what you are doing. Let them know that you will help them learn to take care of themselves and your home together. Ask them what they are thinking about. Rather than asking "why?" focus on where, when, how, and with whom. Lead with curiosity and try to understand more about what excites them. Again, invite them to join you in what you are doing and give them an age-appropriate task. This concept is beautifully described in *Hunt, Gather, Parent* by Michaeleen Doucleff.

> *"When I was raising my children and working full time, it was just easier to do all the household chores without them. I wanted my kids to have fun and not feel badly that they hadn't cleaned up their room. Now that they are grown, I realize that I raised kids who are missing a lot of life skills, like cooking, laundry, managing their money, and even just helping out. I really regret this."*

Teaching children to take care of themselves and the family home is a gift, not a chore. It helps them develop self-confidence. Just lead with a positive point of view, look for the thing they did right, and then show them how to improve the parts that still need to be strengthened without any reprimand; just demonstrate.

Love in the form of touch calms the nervous system, and deep listening provides emotional regulation and empathy. Small children often love cuddling or wrestling. Older kids also might enjoy a backrub or genuine hug just to show that you care.

Exercise

Exercise helps everyone, and it's especially helpful for children and teens with ADHD. It improves memory, attention span, and executive function. Hyperactivity literally calls out for movement; it helps to clear the head of anxious thoughts and gives more room for activating the ability to initiate boring but important tasks. Children should be offered physical play two or three times a day. Being in nature reduces ADHD symptoms.

For students who cannot take stimulant medications, engaging in 10 to 30 minutes of aerobic exercise will increase their focus by up to 45 minutes after exercising.[79] This is why, as an adult, you don't want to spend a lot of time showering and eating after working out. Use that higher productivity time to do harder mental work. When you start fading, eat something and then take a shower.

Routine

Developing a simple, consistent, and predictable routine will greatly reduce stress by creating regular habits that decrease the amount of time spent deciding what to do next. Start by talking with your co-parent about how you would like the day to unfold, and what the ideal start and end time is for the kid(s) and adults. Equipped with those considerations, establish the timing for the day's major events, including preparing for the day, breakfast, transportation to school and work, midday duties, afternoon pickup or activities, homework, dinner preparation, dinner, after-dinner activities, and bedtime. These events should take place at roughly the same time every day. I know that might be an impossible thought, but you'll notice that you and your child will feel calmer and less anxious when both you and they can rely on a consistent schedule.

---

[79] Aylin Mehren, et al., "Physical exercise in attention deficit hyperactivity disorder—evidence and implications for the treatment of borderline personality disorder," *Borderline Personality Disorder and Emotion Dysregulation*, 7 (2020): 1, https://doi.org/10.1186/s40479-019-0115-2.

There are many tricks for making routine chores more interesting. Pair boring activities with interesting ones, like following after-dinner chores with a game or story. Encourage young children to start with any part of the job, such as opening the dishwasher and putting away the silverware. Kids do better when they have a couple of regular jobs that they can comfortably handle. Don't start with feeding the dog; rather, have them play with the dog outside after school or pick up any dirty laundry in their room before they go to bed. Keep three boxes of toys for younger kids and cycle through them, leaving two of them in storage at a time. This keeps them interested in new, yet familiar, objects.

For older kids, involve them in planning the flow of the day. Do they want to share in making lunches or breakfast? Would they rather feed the animals or play with them? Can they meet with you to pick out five outfits for the week on Sunday afternoon? Hang each outfit or have baskets or cubbies to organize the wardrobe for the week ahead. Post a large dry-erase board or a digital calendar in the most used part of the home with everyone's schedule, to help keep your family organized.

We also spoke earlier of the importance of all items having a "home" and the convenience and logic of having a launchpad by the door where each person has a hook and cubby to keep their backpack, sports stuff, shoes, and jacket. Keep your physical space organized in the simplest of designs. Get rid of as much visible clutter as possible. Create a dedicated workspace for homework and a separate place for play.

The way to start your day most successfully is to begin the night before. This means taking a few minutes to plan the next day before heading to bed. It might be more involved if you are also packing lunches or double-checking homework and backpacks, but everything that can be done before sleep in preparation for morning should be done ahead of time. Most of us are familiar with what happens when we wake up late and have to rush through the necessary tasks of getting to school or work on time. Planning ahead enables everyone to follow the morning routine with greater ease and increases the possibility that the family will also get breakfast before walking out the door.

"I realized that I was practicing 'revenge bedtime' more often than I wanted to admit. It was my only time when the house was quiet, and I could watch my shows and not be stressed, but I was averaging five hours of sleep and hated mornings. My kids were always running late and sometimes we all forgot to take our meds. Things felt chaotic. I asked my husband if we could take turns with the bedtime routine and give each other a couple of hours to unwind once we'd completed the after-dinner chores. We then committed to both going to bed by ten. Honestly, I now look forward to reading our mystery novel together, except that one of us usually crashes before the chapter is over. Mornings feel a lot better."

Emotional Regulation

ADHD means having a brain that's wired differently. It's part of who you are, including being a person who feels emotions very deeply and quickly. You may be especially tuned in to how members of your family are feeling, which is both helpful and exhausting. Your child may be exceptionally aware of your emotions as well. Consider being flexible and accommodating. Try to let go of your preconceived notions about how a child of any age is supposed to behave or develop. Instead, pay attention to what your child is actually doing and saying. Ask them what they are feeling and what they might need when addressing their hard feelings.

Parent: "I can see you are upset; are you angry or scared?"

Child: "I'm frustrated!"

Parent: "You are frustrated that you can't go play because I said you had to stay in and finish your homework first?"

Child: "Yeah, it's not fair. Gavin gets to go outside and play basketball."

Parent: "Yes that's true, but he also finished his schoolwork yesterday and today. Do you want to start on your math or your reading first?"

Child: "I don't like doing homework."

Parent: "I know it's often not fun. How about I sit with you and work on my work while you start your math problems?"

Child: "I don't know what to do."

Parent: "Can we look in your backpack and see what you have for math homework?"

Child: "Okay, but how long do I have to do this?"

Parent: "Let's start with 25 minutes, and then we'll take a break for 10 minutes and have some food, and then do a little more after the snack?"

Child: "I wish I could go play."

Parent: "I know, sweetie. Let's see what we can get done in the next bit of time and then there should be time to play outside before dinner."

When we talked about rejection sensitivity, we mentioned the brain feeling like it's flooded with emotions. It feels hijacked by perceived negative feedback, and self-rejection is more painful than for those without ADHD. The self-rejection is often accompanied by feeling that they've disappointed someone. This is where it's so important to practice regulating your own reactions and emotions. The all-important pause before reacting will become your best response. Practice breathing or counting to 20 before responding.

The tone of your response matters more than the words themselves. Stay calm and start by acknowledging how the child feels. If they've done something wrong, remind them of the limit or rule and what they can do next time to improve their effort to meet the goal. They may have made a bad choice, but they are not a bad person.

Here are some examples:

You've been frustrated with your teenager's lack of clean clothes and piles of stuff in the bathroom and their bedroom for the past month. Last weekend, you set them up with their own laundry basket and showed them again how to use the washer and dryer. You did a load of laundry with them and asked that they do their laundry every weekend. Now it's Sunday night and they haven't done any laundry.

Parent: "Michael, hey, it's been great not having any clothes left in the bathroom, and I noticed most of your dirty stuff made it into the laundry basket, but it's Sunday evening and I don't think you did any laundry this weekend. Would you like to set a time in the next couple of days to do another practice run?"

Or with a young child who is learning to make their bed, and you've made it together a few times and now they are doing it alone. You see that all they did was pull the bedspread up over the rumpled sheet and blanket.

Parent: "Susie, that's great that you covered your bed with your bedspread. How does it look to you?"

One of the most critical tenets of learning to be a better parent is to avoid shaming your child. This can be very hard, because most of us were raised in homes where there were strict ideas of what was right and wrong. It is especially challenging if you were dealing with your own troubles with attention and forgetfulness and there were ample opportunities for others to criticize and shame you. Try to begin the conversation with your child by showing them that you are curious about how they feel, not about what they did wrong. Focus on how you are with yourself and your child and less on what you and they are doing.

"When my older son was 13, he babysat my younger son which included making dinner on a gas stove. When I came home, they were both asleep in their beds and the house was in order, but I smelled gas. I stepped into the house and yelled that they needed to get out of the house as soon as possible. We lived in an attached condo and shared walls with two neighbors. I then proceeded to lecture my 13-year-old about the risk that he'd put himself and the neighbors in. I showed him how to turn off the stove properly and again expressed my exasperation with him. At this point, he was totally shut down. It finally dawned on me what he was feeling. I asked him if he was feeling unappreciated. Bingo; tears started flowing. I was able to acknowledge that he'd done a good job feeding and taking care of himself and his brother and just needed to learn more about how to use the stove.

*I also realized I needed to learn more about how to prepare
my 13-year-old to babysit."*

TEACH SKILLS

For most of us, maintaining a positive perspective does not
come naturally. When we are worried about whether our
child is going to make it in the world, we harbor a lot of feelings: anxiety that they won't be able to keep up; anger at the
lack of proper support; resentment that your child demands so
much extra time; or sorrow that the dreams you had for yourself and your child may not be met. Most families are just out-
right exhausted from trying to do all the things necessary to get
through a normal week.

With that backdrop, it can be tough to look for bright spots.
Here's the thing: Your ADHD child sees them instinctively.
Notice the details that bring them joy or have piqued their interest, and then get engaged. They may have serial collections, or a
fascination with an online character, or enjoy a certain genre of
music. Show genuine interest and follow up with questions the
next day. Try to avoid asking questions that sound evaluative or
judgmental, such as questioning what they accomplished, and
focus more on what caught their attention. This might end up
with them providing you a 20-minute retelling of the whole episode of a YouTube video, or it might be that you get to play some
aspect of a game, art, or sport in which they are engaged. Find
something you genuinely like and comment on that. Be careful
with any negative feedback. You know those people who seem
to see the positive in most situations, the glass-half-full folks?
Try to emulate them and practice finding the good things that
accompany the hard things.

Similarly, show passion for your child's skill set, both in personal interests and the life tasks that you hope your child will bring into adulthood. From early on, invite your child to come alongside you as you clean up their room, put laundry in the basket, sweep the floor, load the dishwasher, prepare food, feed the pets, mow the lawn, work on the car, repair the toaster, or go shopping. Not every moment needs to be a teachable moment, but often parents get so overwhelmed that they figure it's just easier to do it themselves. This does not bode well for helping your child learn how to master self-care, money management, care of a vehicle, how to plan, shop, and prepare meals, and what to do when things don't go as planned. Every single skill must be learned; you'll feel closer, and your child will associate you with having taught them things of value. The trick is to meet your child at the developmental level they are at and make the learning fun, or at least not stressful.

ACCESS SUPPORT

Most families have some degree of isolation and are not able to count on a grandparent or uncle or aunt to help raise their kids. If your family lives out of town, consider making weekly video calls and talk about how often you'll be able to see each other. Let your family know that you would value having more contact and the chance for your child to get to know them.

Even if relatives live locally, there may have been rifts or stressors that have made having regular contact with them difficult. I advise making every attempt to invite and include your child's extended family to build a relationship with your child. If you are unable to clear the air by talking things out, consider getting some professional support. Children who have ADHD and have extended family members who demonstrate interest in them are more likely to complete their education. These relationships also are shown to decrease the likelihood that they will suffer from depression, isolation, and mood issues. The tendency in the United States to value individualism over collectivism has led to the deterioration of a strong family foundation and increase in depression and suicide.[80] You may have to actively request more contact and apologize for the ways in which you've contributed to the breakdown in communication. You only have 18 years of raising your child in your home, so if you can mend bridges, I encourage you to do so.

On the other hand, there are families where there simply is too much trauma. If you feel that the degree of abuse or neglect that you suffered in your family of origin was too grave to address and puts you and your child at risk, create a family of choice. Some families adopt aunties and uncles who become very integral to their children's lives. These special friends will give you and your children a deeper sense of community and confidence that you are not alone in the world. These friendships will also teach your children the importance of demonstrating care for people other than immediate family.

Another option might be joining a new parent's group or asking your circle of friends if any of them are interested in having a closer relationship with your child. Kids thrive on having regular contact with caring adults, and you will benefit from being able to count on some consistent time off.

---

[80] Md Talha and Abdulla al Mahmud, *Individualism and Family Breakdown: Examining cultural variation*, (2024), https://www.researchgate.net/publication/380366252_Individualism_and_Family_breakdown_examining_cultural_variation.

Finally, there is a growing body of professionals who are coming to better understand how to support individuals and families with ADHD. Find a prescriber who specializes in working with people with ADHD—if not your pediatrician, then perhaps a psychiatric nurse practitioner, family doctor, physician's assistant, naturopath, or psychiatrist. I also recommend working with a therapist or coach who is knowledgeable and recommended by other people living with ADHD. A skilled professional can have a significant impact on your child's life, helping them and you build skills that you both will use for the rest of your lives.

SELF-CARE

We are back to putting on your oxygen mask first. If you can create a win-win model of caring for yourself and your child, you are teaching them how to take care of themselves. This life skill is best learned early on, not after years of giving everything you have to your kids and then wondering what it is that you truly want.

Take another look at the ideas discussed in Chapter 5. During moments when you feel overwhelmed and self-critical, the best thing you can do for your child is to take care of yourself. Ask for help from another adult to take care of your child and take some time for you. Take care of your body first. Get rest, eat well, and exercise as you like. Do the thing that helps you get in touch with what you are feeling—walking, breathwork, sports, music, art, writing, or talking to a friend. Just find a way to invite your personal expression of deeper feelings.

Once you get clear on what you are feeling, you have a chance to identify your unmet needs. Do you need more support, time alone, community, work changes, or an opportunity to really talk openly with your partner about raising a child with ADHD? When you know what the top-priority need is, ask yourself or someone close to you to address that need. Is it time to make an appointment with a therapist? Do you need to set your alarm for 15 minutes earlier so that you can meditate or exercise a bit before starting the day? You might want to find other families living with ADHD or talk with your boss about accommodations for your own ADHD. Can you ask your partner to sit down with you in the next couple of days and discuss how to better support each other?

Notice the messages you may be telling yourself, such as "I'm too busy to take care of myself," "I need to take care of my kids first, because I feel bad that they are dealing with ADHD," "How can I care for me when there is no time?" or perhaps "All of my resources should go toward my child with ADHD and not to me." Messages like these sabotage your chances of practicing self-care.

Here are some ideas for couples:

- Alternate with your partner putting the kids to bed and/or performing other kid-related jobs, like preparing meals.
- Have a weekly designated time for each of you when you are "off duty."
- Discuss choosing specific entire jobs for yourself, your child, and your partner so that you don't feel like you must do some of everything.
- Take time for yourself, notice how you feel, and then interact with your child and partner after you've done so.

☀ Discuss a self-care budget with your partner, and enjoy feeling valued when you pay for a massage or a night out.

For single parents:

☀ Learn techniques that help you feel calm and loved. Mindfulness meditation is one of the best tools for reaching a state of inner peace. There are other approaches, but finding a quick route to self-regulation is very important when you want to avoid losing your temper or collapsing from fatigue.

☀ Talk to your friends and family about them taking a more active role in your child's life. Knowing that Auntie Helene comes over every Monday afternoon after school and will make dinner gives you a welcome reprieve and your child a chance to receive love from another adult.

☀ Develop parallel play/work to the hilt. Be with your child while they are playing or helping with household chores while you are taking care of your home and meals.

"I tried so many different self-help techniques, and nothing worked for more than a few weeks. I felt so discouraged. After my husband asked me to get evaluated for my own ADHD, I finally realized how many hats I'd been wearing, and the trouble was I was truly the Jill of all trades and the master of none, and I had no idea who I was or what I even wanted anymore. I just wanted to feel more at ease in my life and not exhausted all the time. Once I'd been on Vyvanse for

a couple of months, I realized that I was no longer dreading the dinner hour every evening, and I even had some fun playing games after we did our after-dinner chores. Things felt more normal, and I was so much happier. My kids told me to keep taking my medicine and they would do better with theirs. It was such an eye-opener for my family."

CHAPTER 11 PEARLS

1. Learn everything you can about ADHD.

2. Treat the parent with ADHD first.

3. Evaluate your child ASAP and start medication right away.

4. Broccoli, love, and exercise do matter.

5. Create a daily and weekly routine.

6. Practice emotional regulation techniques; remember to pause before reacting.

7. Teach skills by modeling and giving positive feedback.

8. Ask for and access support from family, friends, and professionals.

9. Practice self-care.

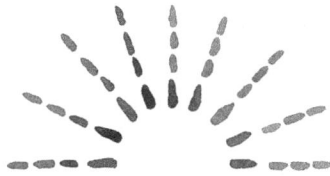

CHAPTER 12

Student Considerations

I'm not sure if my ADHD treatment alone helped with my anxiety or depression. However, it helped in areas that were triggers for them. For example, the anxiety I had around taking tests or timed essays was lessened when I used school accommodations. I was able to enter a test knowing I was in a quiet, controlled room, where I would have enough time for my brain to process and consider questions. This was huge, and I got better grades when I had time to answer all of the questions.

PRESCHOOL AND ELEMENTARY SCHOOL

My experience is largely with teens and adults. If you have younger children, there are experienced experts who can advise you about what is unique and successful for the younger years. It is commonly understood that children with ADHD have trouble controlling their behavior, partly due to problems with impulse control but also because they may have delays in verbal communication skills and will be drawn to stimulation, both positive and negative. Many young kids with ADHD struggle with basic life, social skills, and emotional maturity.

In general, seek out learning environments whose personnel are knowledgeable about ADHD and offer a respectful and supportive classroom for your student. Young kids need a combination of a consistent, structured routine and time to play freely and be creative. They will enjoy expressing themselves in a variety of ways that may require some adjustments to the teacher's instructional style. Teachers who encourage students to learn in different ways might be more supportive of allowing the student with ADHD to get up and move or do art that expresses math concepts, rather than requiring them to sit quietly and write out a solution.

When giving directions to young students, educators do well to make eye contact, give instructions in small batches, and have them repeat those back. Some educators recommend placing kids with ADHD in the middle of the U-shaped classroom seating arrangement, where they will be directly in front of the teacher. If you sit at a rectangular table, ask the child with ADHD to sit at the end of the table opposite the teacher.

Interventions should be offered at the *point of performance.* This means that to teach or give feedback to improve a child's behavior, do it just before the requested performance. If you want a child to help clean up the art table, ask a student who has accomplished this task to show the student with ADHD how to do it, and then have the experienced student accompany the learner the next day and complete the task together. Remind the experienced student to offer only positive feedback. Following a few practices, the student with ADHD can do the task under supervision. When completed, the ADHD student can ask what they forgot, and the other student can show them.

Section 504 under the US Department of Education's Office of Civil Rights ensures that students with disabilities in federally funded schools have equal access to educational opportunities.[81] Among the requirements under Section 504 regulations:

☀ School districts must provide a "free appropriate public education (FAPE) to each qualified student in the school district's jurisdiction who has a disability."

☀ FAPE includes regular or special education, aids, and services to meet the student's individual educational needs.

☀ An appropriate education for a student with a disability could mean education in regular classrooms with or without supplementary services and/or special education as appropriate.

Naturally, public schools are largely underfunded, and teachers often have high student/teacher ratios. This may make the accommodations requested under Section 504 difficult to deliver. You may need to meet privately with your student's teacher and request specific accommodations. Possible accommodations to request:

☀ Seat the child in the front of the class.

☀ Allow them to use fidget toys and/or desk bands that stretch from one desk leg to the opposite side

---

[81] U.S. Department of Education, "Frequently Asked Questions: Section 504 Free Appropriate Public Education (FAPE)," Laws and Policy, updated January 13, 2025, https://www.ed.gov/laws-and-policy/civil-rights-laws/disability-discrimination/disability-discrimination-key-issues/disability-discrimination-providing-free-appropriate-public-education-fape.

(so that the student can move their feet without disrupting others).

☀ Let them get up and walk around or go to a table at the back where they can spend some alone or creative time.

☀ Allow extra time to complete assignments, and/or offer a different testing format.

☀ Provide a quiet space that is less distracting or stimulating to work in.

☀ Give specific instructions on staying organized, like using different colored folders and matching notebooks for each subject.

Under Section 504, if a child must take medications in school, these should be administered by a school representative, not the student or the teacher.

Since teachers are already stressed and under-supported, try to learn what they need, advocate for them, and offer encouragement for what they are doing well.

This bears repeating: Establish clear morning, afternoon, and evening routines. Your child should know what time to wake up, be dressed and in the kitchen, and walk out the door. The main disruptor in the morning is often the parent with undiagnosed or undertreated ADHD. Setting numerous phone alarms and writing out the schedule (or using pictures for younger children) is helpful. Consider placing a large analog clock in every room.

During the second half of the day, the same themes hold true. Anticipating a nutritious snack and some playtime right after school can set a positive tone for the rest of the day.

Having a standard plan for how and when homework is to be tackled will both take the pressure off you and give you permission to help your child start on time. Remember the importance of body doubling; consider sitting with your child and working on your own project while they complete their work. The key is to *get started*.

Bedtime should be a welcome time for comfort, stories, and a final opportunity to connect with your child in a loving fashion. If your child is going to bed on time and has trouble falling asleep, try reading a little longer or playing calming music. Shut down all screen time, including phones, an hour before bedtime. The use of phones is controversial because of all the helpful apps and other resources like music and stories. If you can, go analog at night and leave everyone's phone in a centrally located charging station to discourage an overreliance on screens for entertainment and comfort. Consider using a clock radio and activities like reading or drawing before bed. There are assistive technologies that provide music, such as Google Home and Amazon Alexa devices.

"Being so sensitive to sound meant that I really hated crowds and loud noises. I would often have a lot of anxiety related to this, which led to panic attacks. However, now I know how to prepare myself for the setting, and I can recognize when I feel overstimulated and know how to prevent it from completely overwhelming me. I'm allowed to listen to music when I'm working independently at school."

MIDDLE SCHOOL AND HIGH SCHOOL

Most people with ADHD look back on their middle and high school years with mixed feelings. For many, this is when things start to really fall apart. The difficulties with concentration and memory play out in more noticeable ways when you have multiple classes and overlapping assignments. When you are a person who absorbs others' emotions and has trouble sorting out your own feelings, an environment with many children, lots of noise, and multiple stimuli is overwhelming. Kids with ADHD are generally just trying to survive. They come home hungry and tired, with little interest in engaging with other people or doing homework.

Along with the suggestions regarding routine, diet, exercise, and keeping a positive, loving attitude, what else can help pre-teens and teens feel more comfortable while attending school?

Sleep

A good night's sleep is still the best way to start the day off well. It's best to start when your child is young, model the importance of good bedtime routines, and make their sleeping space a welcome and calming environment. If your teen has developed the habit of staying up late and waking up cranky, first look at your own sleep patterns. If you, too, engage in revenge bedtime—having fun when the house is quiet—you are not likely to be able to help your child get a good night's rest. Talk with your child about how they feel when they get more rest. What can you both do to help them have more nights like that? Take another look at Chapter 9 for sleep recommendations.

I advise setting purposes for times of day: sleep at night, work/study during the day, and play in the evening. This is especially true for high school and college-age students. The goal is to focus on sleep first, being productive second, and completing the day with play, while being unencumbered by anxiety about what you didn't get done. This is the key to feeling great about your day.

Set Up for Success

This includes time management. When your brain operates on "now" and "not now" time, it's hard to think about tomorrow (just another bit of "not now" time). We tend to be more motivated by feelings, so rather than thinking about planning ahead, consider this: "How will I feel in the morning if I have to get everything ready for school after I get out of bed?" If the answer is "anxious" or "frazzled," then try setting a timer for 20 minutes and do some evening preparation to increase your, and your child's, chances for a better day.

Work with your child to create helpful organizational systems at home. (See Chapter 9.) As a reminder: Post a family calendar; establish a launch pad by the front door; set up a dedicated homework space; engage them in meal planning and preparation; set regular start and end times for after-school snacks, homework, and free time; and have everyone in the house help take care of your shared home. Many of my clients have benefited from the 20-minute after-dinner cleanup, where one or two people do the dishes and everyone else randomly grabs a poker chip labeled with a household chore.

School and Homework

Speak to your child's school before classes start to request accommodations and let them know helpful details about your child, including medications, and request access to the online assignment portal. Share the analogy of wearing glasses and supporting their brain to reach its full capacity. ADHD kids are generally highly intelligent and excel when properly supported.

Ask questions about how your kid functions best to help you collaborate to create the environment to support optimal functioning. There may be some surprises: Maybe background noise helps them feel calm or they do better on their homework when they sit in the living room while others are around. They may need soft, comfortable clothing to help them focus, or they might want to do their homework before they leave school. It pays to ask what your child needs to accomplish their work.

Stay interested and in touch with your child, but avoid managing their school experience. Instead, find out more about what excites them, and then help them have more of those opportunities, such as signing up for classes with the most dynamic teachers.

Show your child that you value and prioritize what they care about. This will pave the way for a more open relationship and increase the odds they will tell you when they are struggling academically or personally.

Teen years are a time of big emotions. Teens are sponges who soak up feelings from peers and family. They have an exaggerated tendency to perceive that they have done wrong or are being judged (more so than their absorption of their successes). Try your best to just listen, hear them out, and help them to identify what they are feeling. This opens the door to help them determine what they need and what they, and you, can do to help meet that need.

Help your teenager learn how to self-regulate, giving them possibly the most helpful tool to carry into adulthood.

Youth don't want to be told things, but they do need support in the form of a helpful structure and demonstrations of how to tackle common emotional problems. Teach your kids how to pause, take a breath, and give themselves time to consider a less reactive response to upsetting situations. (You do this, too, right?)

ADHD families endure more stress than other families. Despite the increased ability to hyperfocus and be resilient, creative, and bold, it takes a lot of energy to keep everyone moving forward. This can lead to chronic exhaustion and sap energy, self-esteem, and the ability to show affection. This also generates higher rates of conflict, depression, expenses (for professional support), time needed to complete school, and, sadly, divorce rates as parents neglect their private and social lives, eventually becoming deeply frustrated and anxious.

To combat these negative outcomes, focus on what you have versus what you don't have. Find ways to express thanks daily. Start with an appreciation for your own capacity and love for your child, and you will naturally have more energy and joy in your day. Let your child know specifically how you value them and see their efforts, helping them feel seen and continuing to self-motivate. Teach your kids to write thank-you notes, express gratitude to friends and family, and actively notice goodness in their lives. Not only will this reflect well on them and help them project a positive image, but they will gain positivity in their lives.

Teens with responsibilities at home become more responsible students at school, contributing team members, better classmates, and participants in their school community.

Help them develop empathy and compassion by practicing mindfulness, basic acceptance, and positivity.

"My 15-year-old son was driving me crazy with his back talk and arguing. I was so mad at him that I grabbed a broom and started chasing him around the house. I realized this was nuts and yelled, 'I'm going to my room and don't want to be disturbed. I'll come out when I've calmed down.' When I came out, he had loaded the dishwasher. Maybe timeouts for mom are the best fix."

COLLEGE

Getting ready for college is exciting and overwhelming. Suddenly, all the support from home is gone and you're on your own! No more parents to remind and help you. No more strict schedule. No more teachers who actually know you. It can feel like *too much* freedom. Studies in 2014 showed that only 15 percent of young adults with ADHD held a four-year degree, compared to 48 percent of the control group. Only .06 percent of the ADHD group held a graduate degree, compared to 5.4 percent of the control group.[82]

On the other hand, I have had dozens of college students with ADHD in my practice, and over 90 percent of them have graduated. I also have had many high-level, accomplished professionals, engineers, doctors, nurses, lawyers, CEOs, top strategists, principals, PhD scientists, published authors, head chefs, and many more very effective individuals as clients. Keep those

[82] Aparajita B. Kuriyan, et al., "Young Adult Educational and Vocational Outcomes of Children Diagnosed with ADHD," Journal of Abnormal Child Psychology, 41(1) (2013): 27–41, https://doi.org/10.1007/s10802-012-9658-z.

dreams coming, and yes, set yourself up for success. Proper support with skill building, medicines, and precise use of micronutrients makes a huge difference. Remember that resiliency, adaptability, and being quick learners are some key qualities of people with ADHD. What are some ways to help your student (or you) be most successful at college?

Prepare: In *On Your Own, A College Readiness Guide for Teens with ADHD/LD*, Patricia Quinn, MD, and Theresa Maitland, PhD, ask their readers to complete the College Readiness Checklist, including questions about self-determination, daily living skills, and academic skills.[83]

They suggest that both teens and parents independently complete the scale and then hold a respectful conversation about how they rated their skill levels. Once completed, they suggest making SMART goals together. Where a *vague* goal might be "Go to bed earlier," a corresponding *SMART* goal might be "Be in bed and ready to sleep each school night by 11 p.m." By the way, many employers use SMART goals for their employees, so developing this skill has a bonus benefit.

> **SMART goals**
> Specific, Measurable, Agreed to (or Achievable), Realistic, and Timely. A common metric for building goals.

Action plan: Include **when** you start, **what** you will do, with **which** materials, and **how** you will reach your SMART goal. Evaluate your progress by keeping a written record, chart, or log; even better, accompany that with a buddy check-in. Tell a friend your goal, and agree to have them check in with you in

---

[83] Patricia Quinn and Theresa Maitland, *On Your Own, A College Readiness Guide for Teens with ADHD/LD* (Magination Press, 2011).

a few days to see how you are doing. Once you've checked in and evaluated how you are doing, revise your plan as needed to make it easier to reach your goal. Remember, the R in SMART is for *Realistic*. It is much better to be successful in smaller goals than to fail at bigger ones.

Get coaching: Many college students benefit from having an executive function coach. Lots of students struggle to stay on track in high school and fail to complete assignments on time, despite flexible deadlines, lenient teachers, and attentive parents. Having a coach to help them, especially through the transition period, can be a real asset. A favorite tip one of my college student clients learned from her professor is "Get ahead and stay ahead." When you are prepared for your classes, not only are you less anxious, but you also engage in and enjoy the class material a lot more. Learning can be fun!

Find tips to make life easier: A tip from a client: In a big lecture class with the professor talking from PowerPoints, split your laptop screen and work on that class's homework on one screen while the lecture is on the other screen. This tip came from a college sophomore who managed to get 90 percent of his homework done while in class. Given his 6 a.m. workouts and 3 p.m. football practices, this served him very well. The combination of Adderall and his new study habits brought his GPA up from 1.9 to 3.3 in a year and a half.

Get to know yourself: Quinn and Maitland stress the value of becoming more self-aware. Many people with ADHD are so overstimulated by their environment that they often have difficulty really knowing who they are. They are tired, and when rejection sensitivity overtakes them, it is even more difficult to consider the feedback received from others. There is also a tendency to be somewhat impulsive with interests, often focusing on the likes and dislikes of their friends.

> *"It wasn't until I was in my 50s that I realized that I had serial interests based on the woman I was dating. I bought expensive riding gear because my first girlfriend was into horseback riding. Then, when we broke up, I started developing an interest in scuba diving because the next woman I dated liked that. It wasn't until I fell in love with my yoga teacher that I realized that I really didn't know what I most liked or was good at. Mostly I just wanted to stay home and listen to music, but somehow, I was attracted to dynamic women who were into doing things. I struggled to find my own passion."*

College is a wonderful time to try out various classes and clubs. Take classes taught by popular teachers, but tune in and ask what *you* really like. What feeds your talents, strengths, and interests? It is equally important to recognize your weaknesses and the impact of your ADHD on your ability to succeed in certain kinds of jobs. Hallowell teaches us that people with ADHD will thrive if they can use three principles when deciding what to focus on for work: what you love to do, what you're actually good at doing, and, of course, what you can earn a living doing.[84] Here's one way to visualize this, see Figure 10 on page 190:

---

[84] Edward Hallowell, "5 Rules for Succeeding in the Workplace When You Have ADHD," *ADDitude Magazine*, updated February 16, 2018, https://www.additudemag.com/find-the-right-job-adhd-adults/#:~:text=Your%20job%20ought%20to%20lie,what%20your%20job%20should%20involve.

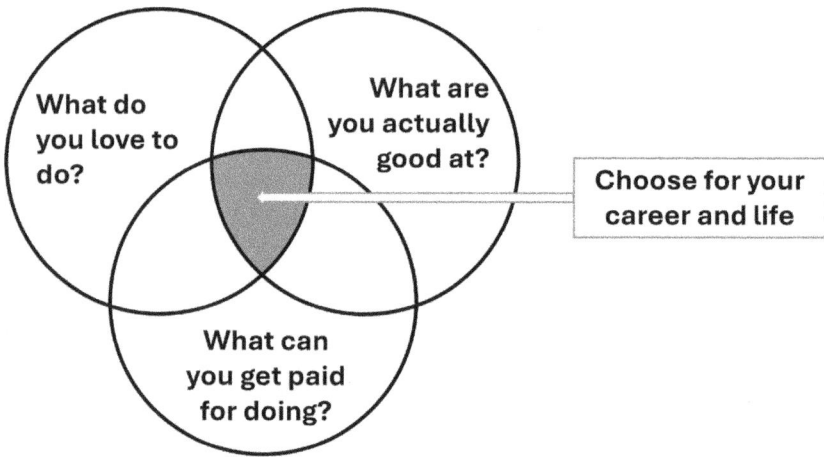

Figure 10. Finding What You Want to Do. Inspired by Edward Hallowell, MD.

You may have no idea what you love, are good at, and what different jobs pay, but college is an excellent time and place to explore the answers to those questions. Decrease the chance of becoming overwhelmed by intense stimulation and set yourself up for success by creating a supportive physical environment and regular routine. Do you want to live with a roommate in a dorm? This is a chance to learn a lot about yourself and make more friends as a freshman. For some students, the need to have a quiet place to retreat to is more important than learning to share space.

How are you going to set up your schedule? Are you a morning person, or do you prefer afternoons? Many of my clients who thrived in college chose classes that met between 10 a.m. and 4 p.m. Generally, people with ADHD need some time to get going in the morning and don't do well with early classes; their energy can fade by midafternoon. Attending class in a block at midday works well for many. Avoid 8 a.m. and evening classes unless you are also working and have no other choice. This is when you'll need an extra dose of stimulant to help you focus into the evening.

It is best to spend your day-times eating, attending class, studying, or exercising, not social-izing or going online for non-school-related activities. Recent research shows that time spent on social media leads to neurocogni-tive inhibitory control difficulties, resulting in a concurrent increase in self-reported impulsive behaviors and a consequent increase in ADHD symptoms in both that and the following year.[85] In simple terms, scrolling on social media shortens your attention span.

> **neurocognitive**
> Relating to or involving cognitive functioning and the associated structures and processes of the central nervous system.

"It wasn't until my junior year that I figured out how to get my homework done. I just didn't hang out with friends until after dinner. I did my schoolwork during the day. At first this was hard, but once I started building this habit, except for the week before finals, I had so much fun in the evenings when a lot of kids were freaking out about deadlines. It was probably the number one thing I felt proud of; I got my work done before dinner. Admittedly I had a few all-nighters in my first years, and those were brutal. It was so nice to be able to relax and play games and music after dinner. I started really enjoying college rather than being anxious all the time about unfinished assignments."

---

[85] Jamina Wallance, et al., "Screen time, impulsivity, neuropsychological functions and their relationship to growth in adolescent attention-deficit/hyperactivity disorder symptoms," *Scientific Reports*, 13 (2023): 18108, https://doi.org/10.1038/s41598-023-44105-7.

Accommodation

You will want to apply for academic accommodations before you arrive at school. Even if it was mentioned in your application, the admissions office is not responsible for arranging accommodations. You need to work with the university's accessibility or disability services office. If you are already in college, go online and read about accommodation requirements. Even if you never use them, it is empowering to know that you can have some extra time on especially challenging assignments and tests and can be granted a priority registration time slot, allowing for better schedule and instructor choice. Note that colleges and universities receiving federal support are legally obligated to provide accommodations for ADHD, but no individualized education plans (IEP) or academic accommodation plans (AAPs) are provided beyond high school. In college, you must ask for help.

You may need a letter from your provider documenting your ADHD diagnosis and describing your treatment. Once the accommodations have been granted, ask for a one-on-one meeting to discuss the available services. Besides extra time on assignments, tests, and priority registration, other services that may be available based on your documented needs include having a note-taker in class, a single dorm room, and software to assist with writing, tutoring, and more.

Upon receiving your accommodation, it is up to you to inform your professors about it at the beginning of the term. You decide if you wish to share your diagnosis of ADHD. This information is confidential. Even if you don't seek or get accommodations, there may be other support, such as study groups or a learning or writing assistance center. Many students struggle with academics in college or have interpersonal challenges with roommates, and there are ways to address those issues. However, if a student also has social anxiety, seeking support may be difficult. Often, students still engage their parents to help advocate, and that is okay, too. Just don't suffer alone.

Sadly, I've seen students struggle with their midterms, not speak up, and then at the last minute withdraw from class to avoid a failing grade. Friends, family, professors, and representatives from the accessibility office all want to help you, but they can't if they don't know you are struggling. You must ask. I'm going to say that again: *You have to ask*. Think about someone you care about coming to you for help. How does that make you feel? It feels good to be trusted and to offer some comfort or advice. Give others the chance to do the same for you.

Social Skills

In addition to setting yourself up for success academically, your college social experience is equally important. It can give you practice talking to new people and building a mental list of conversation starters. People generally enjoy talking about their interests and backgrounds. Come up with more unique ways of asking people about themselves. Some examples: What did they enjoy the most about high school, and do they miss anything? What has surprised them about college? Have they heard about any particularly great professors? Are they planning to explore any subjects they've never taken before? Do they have siblings who went to or are currently in college, too? What facilities at college are they most excited about using—gym, art studio, library, sound studio?

Every college student has periods of loneliness, anxiety, and being overwhelmed. It's very important to recognize when you are not able to self-regulate. When you wake up anxious, go for a run, and still feel sad, or go out with friends and feel alone, it is time to get help. Every school has a health center. Reach out for help as soon as you recognize you are not able to address your own challenges. Many students become isolated and don't tell their friends or family for fear of judgment. They may feel ashamed that they are struggling and think they'll feel better tomorrow or should be able to handle this on their own.

Documentation

One last recommendation to start now and continue into adulthood: Create both paper and digital storage sites that include important documents that you will need over your lifetime. Choose a highly secure storage solution, as the information you are keeping here will include personally identifiable information (PII) that can be used to steal a person's identity. These should include a copy of your birth certificate, Social Security card, driver's license, passport, high school transcript and diploma, and medical documents. In addition, create a separate digital storage space to save information on ADHD that you'll want to refer to or share with others who are interested in you and your ADHD.

CHAPTER 12 PEARLS

1. Create structured environments with routines that support regular movement.

2. Give instructions at the point of performance.

3. Learn about Section 504 benefits available to children with ADHD in federally funded schools.

4. Plan ahead in the evening for the next day.

5. Sleep at night, work/study during the day, and play in the evening.

6. Express interest in what students are doing, not in how much they have accomplished.

7. Practice gratitude for what you do have rather than focusing on what is missing.

8. Work alongside your student and teach them by modeling and giving positive feedback.

9. Get ahead and stay ahead.

10. Practice good self-regulation, and ask for help as soon as you start to falter.

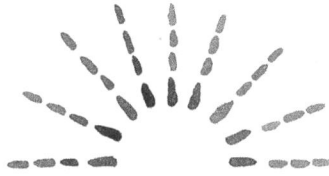

CHAPTER 13

Impact on Relationships

I was so happy for the first months of my relationship with my boyfriend, then we moved in together and things started to change. My housekeeping style is more relaxed. I tend to pick up once a week at the end of the weekend. He wanted things to be tidy each and every day, and he started telling me I was lazy and didn't care about him when I would leave my gym bag on the floor or the mail on the kitchen island. Sometimes I'd find myself interrupting or finishing his sentences for him. Also, it affected our sex life; I was interested, but sometimes by the time we would get into bed, and I had checked my phone and wandered around doing stuff, he'd be asleep; or, if he was awake, then sometimes I'd be too tired or distracted by some worry that was going around in my head. After six months of living together, he told me that it was clear I didn't care about him, and he moved out. I was devastated.

Relationships are challenging regardless of whether one is neurotypical or neurodivergent. People with ADHD struggle with time management, procrastination, prioritization, hyperactivity, and mood dysregulation, all of which can play havoc on a relationship, especially when one or both members of the couple does not understand that these issues can't just be willed away.

It can be confusing to delight in the creative and insightful observations that the partner with ADHD offers, while feeling uncertain about whether they can depend on their partner to remember important details. On the flip side, the person with ADHD will tire of the criticisms and worries being expressed by their detail-oriented mate.

The person without ADHD has trouble understanding why the person with ADHD can't "just do it." Why can't they just pick up their stuff, do the dishes, not leave the tops off containers, pick up the grocery items that were texted to them, and so on. People with ADHD use much of their energy doing the basic things necessary to get themselves up and ready for their day, are often exhausted by late afternoon, and are unable to maintain routine patterns of completing household tasks. They suffer from constantly feeling that they are disappointing their partner, and this adds to their low self-esteem. A person without ADHD may misinterpret their partner's behaviors as proof that they do not care for or respect them and their needs. How does one maximize both people's attributes and take into consideration the forces that create these misinterpretations?

For partners, parents, friends, and co-workers, here are some tips to help you have more success in your relationships with people with ADHD. For those with ADHD, learning these basics will help you accentuate your strengths and address some of your challenges with more knowledge and, ideally, kindness.

"It's okay if learning about ADHD feels overwhelming to you; go easy and gentle on yourself. With that being said, once you are ready to immerse yourself in as much information on ADHD as you can. This will not only help you understand yourself, but it will help you be able to tell loved ones what you need and how your brain works so they can better love and support you."

EDUCATION

Learn as much as you can about how a person with ADHD's brain is wired, so you can understand the attributes and frustrations. Some "easy" tasks can be daunting for someone with ADHD, so ask them to identify which tasks they prefer to take on. For example, they may rather do dishes than laundry. They might be more successful walking the dog than making the bed or vacuuming. Learn when to do certain activities; things requiring more thought should be done earlier in the day. Often people with ADHD struggle to get going in the morning and will have a burst of energy in the evening. Use movement to help stimulate and wake up a sleepy brain, and acknowledge that rest periods and naps can be helpful.

The partner who doesn't have ADHD might be confused by their mate's ability to hyperfocus on something of interest, like a hobby, game, or new pet, but not basic household upkeep. This is often interpreted as the person with ADHD only caring about the "interesting" thing and not the non-ADHD person's important priorities. Understanding that having trouble with executive functioning—getting started and completing tasks after spontaneously getting excited and making a big splash on a new project—can create a lot of frustration for both parties.

The person without ADHD is irritated by the mess and incomplete project or chore. The partner with ADHD feels unappreciated for the effort they put into the part they were hyperfocused on.

Basic household tasks are best addressed by creating specific routines, followed by something fun. Playing dynamic "get stuff done" playlists can really help lift the mood and get people motivated. Select tunes that are uplifting or edgy and not your usual playlist. Your brain will begin to associate these sounds with the urgent need to complete tasks.

If you realize that the person with ADHD may be more likely to come up with creative helpful ideas but will need you, who are without ADHD, to help set up a structure to implement and complete the ideas, things will flow much more smoothly. It may be necessary to have a schedule that changes from time to time to keep you both motivated and working together. Maybe you would enjoy meal planning and cooking together, but grocery shopping is best left to the person without ADHD or done online.

POSITIVE REINFORCEMENT

We all prefer to hear what we've done well. Children with ADHD may hear as many as 20,000 negative remarks by the time they are 10.[86] They expect to be criticized even when the other person is simply stating what they want or need. People with ADHD are especially hard on themselves and benefit from being told

---

[86] Michael S. Jellinek, "Don't Let ADHD Crush Children's Self-Esteem," *Clinical Psychiatry News*, 38 (2010): 12, https://www.thefreelibrary.com/Don%27t+let+ADHD+crush+children%27s+self-esteem.-a0228519256.

what they've done well first and last, with constructive feedback offered in the middle. For example, "It was so nice that you stopped at the store to get food for dinner. I noticed that you also stopped by the drug store, so we didn't get started on making dinner until 8:00. I really like having time with you after dinner and felt sad that the evening was over. Can we try to start making dinner by 6:30 in the future so that we can have our couch cuddle time, too?"

Try asking questions first, rather than stating what you want. For example, you can say, "We talked about doing some chores this weekend. How and when would you like to get started? Which ones are you most interested in doing?" rather than, "You said we'd clean up the yard and take the boxes to Goodwill this weekend. Let's get started at 9 on Saturday. I'll rake the leaves in the front, if you can do the back, so that I can go to the game in the afternoon."

In general, even if you wish you could understand "why" your person with ADHD is doing what they are doing, try to learn more about what they want or what occurred, when something happened or when they would like something to happen, and how they are feeling, as opposed to asking why they did the thing that upset you.

One of my favorite questions is, "What do I need to know to better understand how you are feeling?" When listening to the answer, avoid asking *why*. Ask clarifying questions, such as "When did that happen?" or "What happened after you did the first thing?" or "How do you feel now about what happened?" Avoid giving advice, telling a story about how you had a similar experience, or jumping in to offer support before the person is ready to receive comfort. Remember that people with ADHD are often very accepting and nonjudgmental of others. Try to reflect that in your own response to the person with ADHD.

If the premise of your relationship is that you love and respect each other and demonstrate what you value and appreciate, then it's easier to mutually agree to work on the challenges. Often the person with ADHD will only see their faults, troubles with attending, and impulsiveness in comparison to their organized and punctual partner. They have difficulty recognizing how valuable their creativity, kindness, ability to have fun, and deep empathy are. These attributes are what the non-ADHD member of the partnership fell in love with. To strengthen your bond and bring more joy to your relationship, take time to remind each other what you appreciate about the other.

People with ADHD are great supporters when someone is in crisis. Although the partner without ADHD may feel that the lion's share of supporting falls on their shoulders, it is critical that they are able to be vulnerable and allow their partner with ADHD to support them. When the non-ADHD partner shares their feelings deeply and welcomes their partner's care, they'll have gone a long way toward restoring the balance in the relationship.

> "My partner and friends and I have actual equal and authentic relationships now. When the clouds parted, I was not only able to see myself more clearly, but I was able to see the people around me more clearly as well. I am no longer focused on just the outcomes for them and their feelings, or conversely, just my own feelings. Loving myself first and seeing myself the new way I have learned to allows for more love and compassion in my relationships."

CONNECTION/COMMUNICATION

Knowing that the foundation of ADHD is inattention (i.e., distraction), it can be easy to feel slighted when the person with ADHD is checking their phone, playing a video game, or doing online shopping. Creating a couple of daily ways to check in and connect will help both parties feel seen and loved. Talk about how you each like to be acknowledged in the morning. Is it a hug or quick summary of the day's plans or getting a little exercise together? Similarly, at the end of the day, find a way to come back to mutual communication. Sitting together and rubbing shoulders or listening to one another's rose (positive) and thorn (negative) experience of the day can be very nice. Making sure there's 60 minutes before sleep that's free from electronics, allowing you to be together in some calming way, like reading a story or listening to music, can set the mood for sleep.

When you are thinking about saying something potentially upsetting to your partner, consider if it will cause you both to feel more connected or disconnected. For example, if the dishes have been left undone for days, how will your ADHD partner respond if you say, "I feel like you don't care about me and our home when you leave the dishes for days, especially when I did all of the laundry," versus, "When you did the dishes before bed every night, I felt so happy to walk into a clean kitchen in the morning to make my coffee. How can we get back to that habit?" Then you can wait for a response, and if there's room for a suggestion, you could say, "What if we both do 20 minutes of chores after dinner? I could pick up and do some light cleaning while you do the dishes. Would that work?"

It helps to lead from the perspective that the relationship is constantly growing and deepening. Everyone will have conflict and disappointment as they learn how to improve their communication and feel more connected. If you consider the challenges to be more practice and investment in how much you know and love one another, embracing your errors and practicing how to overcome mistakes will help strengthen your relationship.

Remember to use "I" statements as opposed to "you" statements. For example, "I feel disrespected when I've made dinner and you are not here. I want to feel seen and valued. Would you be willing to talk with me about how to address this by tomorrow?"

Additionally, make sure your requests are specific. The response cannot be, "I promise to do better." It's conceivable that the solution you set up is agreement on a certain number of days a week to share dinner, or that the person with ADHD agrees to do something that their partner values on the nights that they arrive late to dinner. Or maybe the dinner menu could be adjusted to include easy-to-heat meals that the person with ADHD makes on the weekend. On those nights, there is more flexibility for arrival times. Sometimes the issue is not tardiness but rather the lack of advanced notice. The person without ADHD could clarify how much notice they would like if their partner were running late.

Since people with ADHD often hear blame and criticism when that is not what was intended, check if the remark that sent them reeling was, in fact, a criticism. This tendency to hear blame can make it difficult for the non-ADHD partner to express how they are feeling. They may fear that the partner with ADHD will become dysregulated and the person without ADHD may feel like they are not being supported or able to ask their partner for a change. This can lead to burnout and deep discouragement.

When going back to repair a disconnecting interaction, the goal is for both parties to be heard. It can be very challenging for the person with ADHD to move beyond their state of feeling judged and be able to fully attend to their partner. Both people need to be especially aware of the need to pause, breathe, and listen before speaking.

Remember that a person with ADHD brings fresh ideas, spontaneity, positivity, and passion to the relationship. Their challenges with attention to detail and ability to remember (decreased working memory) mean they may miss details that are important to the partner without ADHD. On the upside, people with ADHD tend to not carry grudges and are less likely to be upset with normal errors that people without ADHD may make.

If the non-ADHD partner feels burnt out from doing the important but irregular household tasks like watering the plants, scheduling household maintenance, cleaning out closets, and so on, consider discussing the person with ADHD doing more of the daily chores as part of their everyday routine.

TIME MANAGEMENT

In Chapter 9 we talked about time management strategies. Naturally, this is a major area of stress for couples where one person has ADHD, and more so if you both have ADHD. As a person without ADHD, don't assume your partner with ADHD wants your help managing their time. Ask first and be specific about what it is that helps them feel cared for. Vice versa, people with ADHD may be late because they are doing something to be helpful, like buying flowers for the host. This can be confusing if the non-ADHD person just wants to be somewhere on time. The ADHD person may need some feedback or suggestions as to what makes you feel most loved regarding time management. Which is more important: whether they are clean and dressed or punctual?

When one struggles with executive functioning, it can be difficult to break down a larger task into smaller steps. When you tell a person with ADHD that you want to leave at 4:30, often they will think "no problem" and not consider all the tasks that need to be performed—and the time that will take—before departing. In their mind, they may think, "It'll just take a few minutes to change my clothes and grab my stuff." They might not consider that they have to shower, shave, choose clothing, put on makeup or accessories, and wrap up whatever they were doing in the house. Maybe they also must feed a pet or lock up— all things that take time.

If your partner with ADHD struggles with punctuality, try discussing how much time they typically need to get ready to go to an event. Adding an extra 15 minutes will help decrease anxiety and make getting ready run smoothly. It may be helpful to break down the bigger task into a few smaller steps. If you are leaving at 4:30 to get to a 5:00 event, the person with ADHD may need to tell themself to be ready to leave by 4:15. Their plan could be setting a reminder for getting in the shower at 3:30, being dressed and made up by 4:00, and wrapping up final details before walking out the door by 4:15. Do not assume they will think ahead about all the steps they need to take to leave on time. Ask them how they would like to be supported. Do they want a personal reminder, or do they prefer alarms? Do they need more than one alarm?

Lists can be very helpful. When you create a deadline for departure or completion of a project, also create a checklist for each of the action steps. This helps train your ADHD brain to realize that you need to start getting ready 45 minutes before departure if you need to shower before leaving. This can also be helpful for common multistep household tasks, like laundry, dishes, or cleaning the bathroom. Some people like using a printed checklist when they first practice being more punctual or successful when executing a boring task.

It helps to recognize that *punctuality is a personal choice*, and the person with ADHD may not care as much about this value. They may recognize that there are certain events that you can't be late for, like professional meetings or appointments with your doctor or therapist. The urgency around these types of commitments will likely help them be on time. If the person without ADHD feels that they don't want to accommodate their ADHD partner's tardiness, they can suggest providing their partner a 15-, 5-, and 2-minute warning. If negotiated ahead of time, and the ADHD person is not ready, the person without ADHD would be permitted to go on their own to avoid blaming their partner for being late. Be sure to say goodbye and not just storm off.

Try not to take the ADHD person's behavior personally. Recognize that the person with ADHD is not intentionally disrespecting you, their partner. This is a bona fide part of their neuronal circuitry. People with ADHD are remarkably nonjudgmental and accepting. Knowing this can provide additional ways of addressing such challenges.

Remember that the non-ADHD partner is not responsible for the ADHD partner getting to work, or the gym, or any other non-shared function, on time. With their permission, help the person with ADHD set up apps, a shared calendar, timers, or alarms, and then acknowledge when things go well to help create a system of mutual support.

Consider these tips when trying to build a new habit:

☀ Attach the task to something you are already doing on a regular basis, like taking your supplements right before you brush your teeth or take your medicine.

☀ Take advantage of your phone or digital assistant to set alarms. Try using special ring tones: first warning—lighter music/tone; second warning— more urgent music/tone; third warning—something very unpleasant and harsh that you might want to turn off before it rings. Train your brain to recognize the "ready, set, go" message signaled by the three alarms.

☀ Give yourself a minor consequence that hurts a little if you fail your own alarm system; e.g., you must make a small contribution to your favorite charity.

- Be sure the consequence is you doing something positive for someone else, rather than a personal punishment.

If I could offer just one tip for you to address your issues with completing tasks, it would be to use a **list**. Use a single notebook. When you write down a task, limit it to things that you really need/want to get done in the next two days. Write long-term tasks in the center fold of the notebook and check them periodically. When you finish the day, start a new list, carrying incomplete items over from the previous day. You should only operate from two pages: a personal and a work list. Keep the old pages to look back, gain a sense of accomplishment, and help you to perfect your list-making skills.

Following on the heels of that tip, write your top three tasks on a colored 3x5-inch index card the night before, and think about which of those things you are going to do first. People who do the hardest thing first—like sending an email they've been putting off—find that they then sail through the subsequent tasks. If you can't start with the hardest one, it's okay; just start with any task first and build up your skills.

"I used to beat myself up when my partner told me I had interrupted him again and asked why I couldn't just listen. He said I clearly didn't care enough and was only interested in myself. Now, when I feel something is urgent to say, I count to five and then ask him if I can share my thoughts. Now he knows that what I'm going to say is important to me. When I'm done, he says, 'Can I tell you what matters to me?' and I am more ready to listen. That way we both get to talk and listen. It feels more even now."

EMOTIONAL REGULATION/REJECTION SENSITIVE DYSPHORIA

People with ADHD have very strong emotions. They may experience greater highs, joy, exhilaration, and excitement. Conversely, their downs can include intense feelings of anger, disappointment, and self-criticism. Knowing that you or your partner is prone to more extreme emotions can be helpful when the negative ones show up. It helps to not take these expressions personally and to accept that they are often exaggerated due to the person with ADHD's more sensitive nervous system.

Since their own perception may be that they are wrong or bad or not lovable, much of their negativity is directed at themselves. This can be hard to recognize when they are pushing you away or having trouble expressing themselves clearly.

Generally, using good listening skills, such as asking for more details about what happened and how they are feeling, rather than defending yourself or telling them how their behavior makes you feel, works best to return to a more even keel. Once the person with ADHD feels reassured of your love and can express their hurt and anger, there will be more of an opening for you to talk about your feelings.

Some couples find that they may want to have two separate conversations. The first one supports the person with ADHD expressing themselves, while the non-ADHD partner listens and learns more about what their partner is experiencing. Once the ADHD person feels calmer and less dysregulated, then the person without ADHD will find that their feelings are more likely to be heard and understood by their partner with ADHD.

Regardless of whether you have ADHD, finding ways to regulate your emotions before you say or do something you'll later regret is a necessary skill. When you start feeling upset, the trick is to recognize that things may be escalating and need intervention. Hopefully, initially, it will just be a minor adjustment to pause and take some deep breaths. If you feel you are at risk of getting angry, try literally stepping away from the stimulus that makes you feel upset. Removing yourself physically and moving to a different, calmer place will help regulate your emotions.

Sometimes our "brakes" fail us when our brain goes super-fast. Our executive functioning doesn't work well when we have strong emotions. When this happens and we hurt each other, it is important to do repair work and mend the relationship. Acknowledge your own error, and own the fact that you may have misinterpreted your partner's behavior or misjudged the importance of a request or deadline. If each person can take ownership for their part in the problem, not judging the other and listening carefully to what their partner is feeling, healing will occur. Once a clear description of how you are feeling is shared and openly received and acknowledged by both parties, you have an opportunity to recognize your own fears and more deeply know your partner. This vulnerability promotes intimacy.

"I have learned a lot about how ADHD can affect conversation. When I'm conversing and upset, I feel like I need to get a point out at that moment, and if I don't, it is all I am thinking about and I am not actively listening. I have been more personally aware of the value of listening and not always having to put my input/experience into every conversation, even if that is all that I am thinking. Now, I still feel it's urgent, but I can pause and know I need to ask my partner if they can listen to me first."

GRATITUDE

The ADHD brain craves dopamine, so it is especially important for the person with ADHD to hear thanks. This gratitude will help fuel their ability to keep working on necessary, but often boring, tasks. If the person without ADHD does not necessarily need praise or appreciation to complete basic household tasks, they may not realize that their ADHD partner does.

Celebrate small successes or acknowledge the "roses" (and not just complain about the "thorns") to bring more energy and joy back into the relationship.

Sometimes just expressing thanks for the smallest consideration can make the whole day better, like saying, "Thanks for letting the dogs out so that I could sleep a little longer," "I noticed you put out the recycling," "That meal last night was so tasty," "I love it when you rub my shoulders before I fall asleep," and "I appreciate when you told me you didn't like how I interrupted you—it makes me want to pause before I speak."

Acknowledge the small ways in which you appreciate each other. One of you may be better at planning, and the other can pack the car quickly and efficiently. One may enjoy thinking through the details of a beautiful meal, while the other might be a one-person whirling cleanup crew. Specific compliments feel better than a general remark. Try something like, "Thanks for writing down my grocery list request and remembering to pick it up after work. I know that it takes some effort to remember everything. I really appreciate you doing that." As opposed to, "Thanks for stopping at the store."

Whenever possible, try to phrase feedback with praise for what you like or is working, as opposed to criticism for what you don't like or want. The ADHD brain is looking for the reward and is easily triggered by negative remarks. This can be especially difficult for people who tend to value truth first. The problem is that people cannot hear the truth if it is delivered in an unloving manner. Equally, love without truth is not love.

People with ADHD often have a great sense of humor and love games. If you can make a chore into a game or challenge, it will be much more likely to be completed. This aligns with playing upbeat music while engaged in the task or enjoying a treat when done. ADHD people like more immediate rewards that don't have to be big or expensive. A hug or something enjoyable to eat are good options, as is playing a game together or watching another episode of a favorite show.

SEX

Sex can be challenging when living with lots of distraction, mental hyperactivity, and fatigue. I suggest talking about what you both enjoy, using when, what, and how questions. When do you like having sex—in the evening, daytime, planned, or unplanned—and how often? What do you enjoy in terms of emotional and physical expressions of love? Talk about foreplay and arousal, music, setting, nudity, and toys. Ask each other how you like to be touched and consider coming up with some nonverbal cues that indicate you'd like to make love (or stop).

Women often need more emotional connection *before* having sex than men, who are more likely to feel more emotionally connected *by* having sex. Naturally, this is not true for everyone—there are certainly many women who enjoy "just being physical" and men who love to talk first and play second. Explore what your partner prefers.

A word about distraction: If you are having trouble focusing, consider what helps you focus before making love. Yes, it might be medication or caffeine, but it also might be to set aside time for sex when you are not exhausted. Planning to spend Sunday mornings together or even taking an occasional mental health day can be wonderful.

At the end of overwhelming days, check in with your partner with a back or foot rub, head scratch, and some gentle connection before sleep. You will both feel closer and rest better.

DON'T SWEAT THE SMALL STUFF

Have you made a nice meal only to have your partner comment on the messy kitchen? Are you annoyed by your partner noticing the spot on your outfit rather than how nice you look in it? Do you find yourself getting caught up with some details that you perceive to be critical of you when others don't experience it the same way? If you want to thrive, the importance of being here now and focusing on what is valuable and beautiful will serve you well.

Many religious and philosophical teachings focus on the importance of loving without judgment. How can we accept one another just the way we are? Loving someone with ADHD can be a tremendous boost for those who struggle with placing excess emphasis on productivity and order and are less able to "be here now," enjoying what is right in front of us. Some have described it as bringing childlike joy and innocence back to a relationship. Relationships that have grown stale may lack a sense of wonder, magic, and spontaneity. In addition, the flow of fresh, out-of-the-box ideas and the ability to multitask and hyperfocus on urgent tasks can be a real advantage.

In *Trusting the Gold*, Tara Brach beautifully describes the concept of "this is it." Essentially, this moment right here, right now, is all we have. Why not enjoy and soak it up, no matter the experience? Just feel it deeply and recognize how alive and human we each are. We get to choose how we interpret this one moment. Do we hold onto our disappointment? Or do we let the small things go and cherish the larger truths of love, respect, and meaning?[87]

People with ADHD are deeply sensitive and loving. They can come up with new ideas that others can't imagine, helping them develop a greater sense of confidence. They are people who will go the extra mile to help someone less fortunate. Yes, they are also the people who often show up late and struggle with common, boring tasks. If, as a couple, you can both acknowledge the person with ADHD's challenges with organizational and time management skills, along with valuing their many attributes, there is less likelihood of shaming or blaming.

The key here is to come from a positive perspective. What skills do you bring to the relationship? How do you complement and balance each other? Are there differences that you choose to acknowledge and capitalize on, and are there tasks that are better hired out or done together because you agree that neither of you like cleaning the bathroom or mowing the lawn?

All couples have communication issues. Be careful not to blame the partner with ADHD for all the problems. Generally, people with ADHD are very perceptive and will pick up on issues that are, in fact, problematic in their partner's communication style. If each of you regularly feel unheard or blamed, you need some support in the form of couple's therapy. While searching for a therapist, many of my clients have found some success in the following approach from Marshal Rosenberg's Nonviolent Communication.[88]

---

[87] Tara Brach, *Trusting the Gold* (Sounds True Publishing, 2021).
[88] Rosenberg, *Nonviolent Communication*.

When things fall apart and you are sad, angry, or feel lost:

1. Offer yourself empathy for what you are feeling, without judgment. Examples: acknowledging that you feel scared, alone, unworthy, hurt, or lost.

2. Figure out exactly what the deep-down feeling is. Remember that anger is generally a cover for hurt, fear, or loss.

3. Identify the "unmet need" associated with the feeling. If you are frightened, then the unmet need might be to feel safe.

4. Make a doable request of yourself or your partner that will help meet the unmet need. Ask for a specific time in the next day or two to talk about how to create more safety.

To put it into practice: Say you have an argument about being punctual to a friend's dinner invitation. The person with ADHD spent a little extra time before coming home to pick up a special bouquet of flowers that she knows their friends will really love. Her coming home later than expected has now made you late for the party. You are frustrated and say, "You always do this, and I just told you last week that I really want to be on time to this dinner." She says, "I just wanted to get them something special since they really love dahlias, and they are in season right now." You leave for the party 30 minutes late; neither of you speak to the other on the way to the party, and you both feel out of sorts all evening. On the way home, she says, "I'm sorry I was late, honey; can we let this go?" You say, "No, I'm tired of not being respected. It seems like your tardiness always makes me late. You know it's important to me, and you just don't care about me."

If she was practicing nonviolent communication, she might think: "I'm hurt that my partner is angry with me, and it's hard to want to take care of my friends, my partner, and me all at the same time. I feel scared that they see me as being broken and maybe not lovable. My need to feel valued is not being met. I'm wondering if we could set time aside in the next couple of days to talk about what they value in me."

The partner's nonviolent communication might include, "I'm hurt that my wife is so inconsiderate of my feelings. I'm afraid that I don't matter to her. I feel scared that she really doesn't love me or understand how important it is for me to be on time with friends. My need to feel secure in my experience of her acting in loving ways is not being met. I'd like to ask her to talk this weekend about whether she'd be willing to discuss a way to be more punctual when we have commitments to other people." As previously mentioned, these are the tenants of Marshall Rosenberg's teachings about Nonviolent Communication. Check him out online or read his book *Nonviolent Communication* listed in the bibliography for more information.

In addition to identifying the root feeling, unmet need, and doable request, use "I" statements and speak of your own experience, rather than describing the other person's. Also, listen for the root or core feeling that underlies those angry outbursts. Give the person who is describing their experience plenty of time to really identify their feelings. When your partner starts expressing how they are feeling, consider saying, "Tell me more."

Often, it works best for one person to speak and the other to just listen and maybe ask clarifying questions. Check in with the speaker to be sure they are done, then paraphrase what they've said to confirm that you truly understand their sentiments. Once the speaker has fully identified and shared their experience, the listener has the opportunity to share theirs. You may need to have two separate conversations.

Be accountable for your part of the problem, even if you don't understand why you said or did something; acknowledging that you contributed to the disconnection will help diffuse the tension. If you start by owning your part and then offering to work on repairing the rift by better understanding how your behavior started and what you might do to get your needs met ahead of time, you just may prevent future blow-ups or at least learn how to address them more quickly when they arise.

The most important takeaway about ADHD and relationships is that *you are in a relationship.* By this, I mean there are two people, each with equal value and responsibility for the relationship. The person with ADHD is not the patient or the child. The person without ADHD is not the fixer or the parent. You each chose to be in this dynamic, creative, and often fun relationship. You each choose to be with a person who experiences the world differently from you. Find ways to capitalize on it, enjoy your differences, and help each other with your individual challenges. Can you agree to some routines that support your home and relationship and be open to spontaneous mini adventures? Can you show appreciation for the unique ways in which your partner expresses their love for you?

> *"I feel better connected. I feel more present. And the relationships have improved in quality. I think it makes me understand my behavior more. I am able to better express myself and my thought process. I am able to think before I speak most of the time."*

"Getting treated for ADHD has had a very positive impact. I'm able to make better friends and communicate my needs better. Feeling more in control of my own life is helping me feel more able to open up to friends and family and genuinely enjoy my life."

"ADHD treatment has had a huge positive impact on my relationships. My husband and I are more easily able to talk about differences in how we operate and better understand how the other person works. We're more forgiving with each other now that we know how differently the other person thinks and works. I'm more patient with my children. I try to embrace their pace and gently bring them back on task when they get distracted. I make sure they're in charge of their own space and help them bring about order when needed. I'm also very aware that they may have ADHD and experience RSD, so I try to encourage process over perfection and ensure they always feel loved and accepted."

CHAPTER 13 PEARLS

1. Divide up household tasks based on what you like doing, and be fully responsible for the complete task.

2. Offer each other positive reinforcement, and notice what has been completed, as opposed to what is not done.

3. Pause and assess whether what you're about to say or do is going to result in connection or disconnection.

4. Always plan extra time, and break tasks down into 20- to 30-minute parts.

5. When feeling upset, have the person with ADHD express their feelings first, and have the partner just listen and reflect back what they've heard. Then switch and repeat.

6. Express gratitude for aspects of each other's personality in a demonstration of your love.

7. Make fun and sex a priority. Talk about when, what, and how to meet both of your needs.

8. Seek couple counseling if you can't readily find a way to make positive progress alone.

9. Don't sweat the small stuff. Cherish the larger truths of love, respect, and meaning.

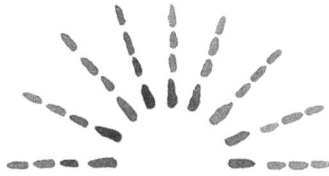

Afterword

Dear person with ADHD, or person who is helping someone with ADHD,

Thank you ever so much for reading this book! I thought it might be helpful to collect the key points to take away from the book:

☀ **ADHD is real**. It presents in a myriad of ways.

- Most of the *Winnie the Pooh* characters have ADHD. Yes, some are hyperactive (think Tigger and Piglet) while others are dreamy (Winnie the Pooh), others are irritable or depressed (Rabbit and Eeyore), and some have wisdom and oversight (Owl). Remarkably, they are all lovable and look out for one another.

- Yes, forgetfulness and having trouble getting started are hallmarks of this brain type. You'll also discover enormous creativity, kindness, and empathy for others.

- Even if you don't appear hyperactive, you'll notice your brain goes a lot faster than the brains of people without ADHD. Great ideas may be generated—or maybe you are just running in circles and getting exhausted.

☀ Few have heard of **rejection sensitivity**, but it well describes ADHD's least known characteristic: extreme emotional sensitivity to the perception of being rejected, criticized, or teased.

☀ Your **genetics and lab values** can guide you to choose the best medication and micronutrients. Consider having genetic and laboratory testing done or offering it to your patients. There's more to discover when testing for biochemical imbalances that impact your mental and physical health.

- Test, don't guess, and then address the deficiencies with quality nutrients, minerals, vitamins, and other micronutrients.

☀ Start with **trialing stimulant medication**. Begin low and go slow, but try them, first and foremost. Do not start with antidepressants or supplements.

- Help your brain's neurotransmitters step into action and then make the other necessary changes, such as incorporating nutrients, taking supplements, practicing mindfulness, and doing exercise, to improve your health and well-being.

☀ **Everything has a place**, and every task deserves to be written in your **To-Do List Notebook**—just one place for things and ideas.

- If the job is not urgent, then make yourself accountable to another person, ask for help in confirming that you've completed the task, or even use a "body double."

☀ **Girls and women** are often misdiagnosed as having anxiety and depression when the underlying condition is ADHD. They also have hormones that impact how they metabolize medication and may need adjustments based on their cycle.

- They are particularly impacted by discrimination at work and should access the **Job Accommodation Network** for support (see Helpful Resources).

☀ **Parents**, remember that ADHD is genetic, and odds are high that one or both of a child's biological parents have it. Get yourself treated first and then have your child evaluated. If your child is nonbiological, work extra hard at learning about this genetic condition.

- Bookend your day with a morning and evening routine that assures that you and your child's needs are both met.

- Model daily activities of living and include positive feedback.

- Take care of yourself and ask for help from family, friends, and professionals.

☀ **Students** should apply for accommodations from their schools.

- Create purpose for times of the day: sleep at night, work during the day, and play in the evening.

- Younger children need a variety of engaging learning environments.

- Practice creating and completing SMART goals.

☀ **Couples**, educate yourselves about what ADHD is and isn't.

- Express appreciation for what you value in each other.

- Don't sweat the small stuff.

- Create systems that support both of you and allow room for plenty of fun and intimacy.

Now, start your own journey. Find a skilled practitioner, and if you can't, ask your primary care provider if they are open to learning more about how to treat ADHD. Download helpful handouts from my website to bring to your clinician. If you are a doctor, nurse practitioner, or physician assistant who would like to learn more, contact me directly and I'll share some options.

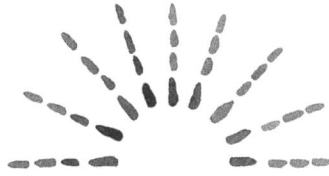

Helpful Resources for ADHD

NATIONAL ADHD ORGANIZATIONS (US)

ORGANIZATION	WEBSITE
ADD Coach Academy	www.addca.com
ADDitude Magazine	www.additudemag.com
ADDiva—Women and ADHD	addiva.net/
ADHD & You	www.adhdandyou.co.uk
ADHD Evidence Project (Stephen Faraone, PhD)	www.ADHDEvidence.org
American Academy of Child Adolescent Psychiatry ADHD Resource Center	www.aacap.org/aacap/families_and_youth/resource_centers/adhd_resource_center/Home.aspx
The American Professional Society of ADHD and Related Disorders (APSARD)	www.apsard.org
American Psychiatric Association	www.psychiatry.org
Attention Deficit Disorder Association	www.add.org

ORGANIZATION	WEBSITE
Best Value Schools—Guide for Students with Learning Disabilities	https://www.bestvalueschools.com/guide-for-students-with-learning-disabilities/
Children and Adults with Attention-Deficit/ Hyperactivity Disorder (CHADD)	www.chadd.org
How to ADHD	https://howtoadhd.com/ youtube.com/howtoadhd
National Alliance on Mental Illness (NAMI)	https://www.nami.org/about-mental-illness/mental-health-conditions/adhd/
National Resource Center on ADHD (NRC) (a program of CHADD)	https://chadd.org/about/about-nrc/

INTERNATIONAL ADHD ORGANIZATIONS

ORGANIZATION	WEBSITE
ADHD Ireland	www.adhdireland.ie
ADHD New Zealand	www.adhd.org.nz
ADHD Support Australia	www.adhdsupportaustralia.com.au/
ADHD World Federation	www.adhd-federation.org/
Attention Deficit Disorder Information and Support Service	www.addiss.co.uk
Australasian ADHD Professionals Association	aadpa.com.au/
Centre for ADHD Awareness, Canada	www.caddac.ca

INTERNATIONAL ADHD PRACTICE GUIDELINES

PUBLICATION	WEBSITE
Australian: AADPA	adhdguideline.aadpa.com.au/
Canadian: CADDRA	adhdlearn.caddra.ca/ wp-content/uploads/2022/08/ Canadian-ADHD-Practice-Guidelines-4.1-January-6-2021.pdf
United Kingdom: NICE	www.nice.org.uk/guidance/ ng87/

RECOMMENDED READING

A New Understanding of ADHD in Children and Adults, 1st Edition by Brown, Thomas E., PhD (Routledge, 2013).

A Radical Guide for Women with ADHD: Embrace Neurodiversity, Live Boldly, and Break Through by Solden, Sari, MS, and Michelle Frank, PsyD (New Harbinger Publications, 2019).

ADHD 2.0: New Science and Essential Strategies for Thriving with Distraction—from Childhood Through Adulthood by Hallowell, Edward M., MD, and John J. Ratey, MD (Ballantine Books, 2021).

ADHD and Asperger Syndrome in Smart Kids and Adults, 1st Edition by Brown, Thomas E., PhD (Routledge, 2021).

ADHD & Us: A Couple's Guide to Loving and Living With Adult ADHD by Robertson, Anita LCSW (Callisto, 2020).

Adult ADHD: Diagnostic Assessment and Treatment, 4th Edition by Kooij, J. J. Sandra MD, PhD (Springer, 2022).

Divergent Mind: Thriving in a World That Wasn't Designed For You by Nerenberg, Jenara (Harper Collins, 2020).

Driven to Distraction (Revised): Recognizing and Coping with Attention Deficit Disorder by Hallowell, Edward, MD, and John Ratey, MD (Anchor Books, 2011).

Finally Focused: The Breakthrough Natural Treatment Plan for ADHD That Restores Attention, Minimizes Hyperactivity, and Helps Eliminate Drug Side Effects by Greenblatt, James, MD, and Bill Gottlieb CHC (Harmony, 2017).

How to ADHD: An Insider's Guide to Working with Your Brain (Not Against It) by McCabe, Jessica (Rodale, 2024).

Hunt, Gather, Parent: What Ancient Cultures Can Teach Us About the Lost Art of Raising Happy, Helpful Little Humans by Doucleff, Michaeleen (Avid Reader Press, 2021).

Integrative Therapies for Depression: Redefining Models for Assessment, Treatment and Prevention, First Edition by Greenblatt, James, MD, and Kelly Brogan, MD (CRC Press, 2021).

Taking Charge of ADHD: The Complete, Authoritative Guide for Parents, Fourth Edition by Barkley, Russell, PhD (Guilford Press, 2020).

Thriving with ADHD Workbook for Kids: 60 Fun Activities to Help Children Self-Regulate, Focus, and Succeed by Miller, Kelli LCSW MSW (Althea Press, 2018).

Understanding Girls with ADHD: How They Feel and Why They Do What They Do by Nadeau, Kathleen G. PhD, Ellen B. Littman PhD, Patricia O. Quinn, MD (Advantage Books, 2020).

Your Brain's Not Broken: Strategies for Navigating Your Emotions and Life with ADHD – For Neurodivergent Men and Women or Parents of ADHD Children by Rosier, Tamara PhD (Revell Books, 2021).

RECOGNIZED ADHD EXPERTS

ADHD EXPERT	WEBSITE
William (Bill) Dodson, MD, LF-APA	https://www.dodsonadhdtreatment.com/
James Greenblatt, MD	https://www.jamesgreenblattmd.com/
Edward (Ned) Hallowell, MD	www.drhallowell.com
Sandra Kooij, PhD	https://www.eunetworkadultadhd.com/author/sandra-kooij/
Ellen Littman, PhD	https://www.drellenlittman.com/
Terry Matlen, LMSW, ACSW	https://www.understood.org/en/people/terry-matlen
Kathleen Nadeau, PhD	https://thechesapeakecenter.com/our-founder
John Ratey, MD	www.johnratey.com
Ari Tuckman, PsyD, MBA	https://adultadhdbook.com/

ADDITIONAL SUPPORT

ORGANIZATION/ INDIVIDUAL	PURPOSE	WEBSITE
Ann Hathaway, MD	Expert in cognitive decline, bio-identical hormone therapy, and functional medicine	https://annhathawaymd.com/
The Center for Nonviolent Communications	International peacemaking organization specializing in resolving differences through dialogue	www.cnvc.org

ORGANIZATION/ INDIVIDUAL	PURPOSE	WEBSITE
Find a Helpline	Locate crisis assistance for a variety of topics, including suicide and domestic violence	www.findahelpline. com
The Institute for Functional Medicine	Information about functional medicine for practitioners and others	https://www.ifm. org/
Job Accommodation Network	Provides employers with job accommodation solutions, strategies, and guidance on the ADA	www.askjan.org
Speaking Grief	Support for those dealing with the loss of a family member	www.speakinggrief. org

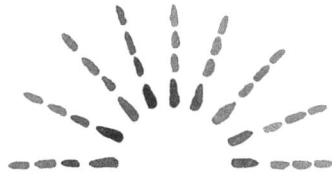

Bibliography

ADDA Editorial Team. "Impact of ADHD at Work." ADDA.org. 2023. https://add.org/impact-of-adhd-at-work/.

ADHD Evidence Project. "Are There Positive Aspects to ADHD?" ADHDEvidence.org. 2022. https://www.adhdevidence.org/blog/are-there-positiveaspects-to-adhd-2.

ADHD Evidence Project. "Get to know ADHD." ADHDEvidence.org. Accessed June 5, 2025. https://www.adhdevidence.org/.

ADHD+ Support. "Famous People with ADHD/AS." ADHD-Support.org.uk. Accessed August 4, 2025. https://adhd-support.org.uk/famous.htm.

Advokat, Claire, and Mindy Scheithauer. "Attention-deficit hyper-activity disorder (ADHD) stimulant medications as cognitive enhancers." *Frontiers in Neuroscience* 7 (2013): 82. https://doi.org/10.3389/fnins.2013.00082.

Amen, Daniel. *Healing ADD: The Breakthrough Program that Allows You to See and Heal the 6 Types of ADD*. Berkley Publishing Group, 2001.

American Academy of Family Practice. *ADHD in Children and Adolescents*, Endorsed, April 2020. https://www.aafp.org/family-physician/patient-care/clinical-recommendations/all-clinical-recommendations/ADHD.html.

American Psychiatric Association, ed. *Diagnostic and Statistical Manual of Mental Disorders, Fifth Edition, Text Revision (DSM-5-TR)*. American Psychiatric Publishing Inc., 2022.

Attention Deficit Disorder Association. "Adult ADHD Questionnaire: Self-Report Scale (ASRS-V1.1)." ADD.org. Accessed July 14, 2025. https://add.org/wp-content/uploads/2015/03/adhd-questionnaire-ASRS111.pdf.

Australian ADHD Guideline Development Group. *Australian Evidence-Based Clinical Guideline for Attention Deficit Hyperactivity Disorder (ADHD), First Edition*. AADPA.com. 2022. https://aadpa.com.au/guideline/.

Barkley, Russell. "How ADHD Affects Life Expectancy." *ADDitude Magazine*. Updated March 25, 2025. https://www.additudemag.com/adhd-life-expectancy-video/.

Barkley, Russell A., Kevin R. Murphy, and Mariellen Fischer. *ADHD in Adults: What the Science Says*. Guilford Press, 2010.

Biederman, Joseph, and Stephen V. Faraone. "The effects of attention-deficit/hyperactivity disorder on employment and household income." *Medscape General Medicine* 8, no. 3 (2006): 12. https://pubmed.ncbi.nlm.nih.gov/17406154/.

Blum, Kenneth, Amanda Lih-Chuan Chen, Eric R. Braverman, et al. "Attention-deficit-hyperactivity disorder and reward deficiency syndrome." *Neuropsychiatric Disease and Treatment* 4, no. 5 (2008): 893–917. https://doi.org/10.2147/NDT.S2627.

Boot, Nathalie, Barbara Nevicka, and Matthijs Baas. "Creativity in ADHD: Goal-Directed Motivation and Domain Specificity." *Journal of Attention Disorders* 24, no. 13 (2017): 1857–1866. https://doi.org/10.1177/1087054717727352.

Brach, Tara. *Trusting the Gold*. Sounds True Publishing, 2021.

Brattberg, Gunilla. "PTSD and ADHD: Underlying factors in many cases of burnout." *Stress and Health* 22, no. 5 (2006): 305–313. https://doi.org/10.1002/smi.1112.

Brown, Thomas E. "The Brown Model of Executive Function Impairments in ADHD." BrownADHDClinic.com. Accessed June 7, 2025. https://www.brownadhdclinic.com/brown-ef-model-adhd.

Cagnacci, Angelo and Martina Venier. "The Controversial History of Hormone Replacement Therapy." *Medicina* 55, no. 9 (2019): 602. https://doi.org/10.3390/medicina55090602.

Canadian Attention Deficit Hyperactivity Disorder Resource Alliance (CADDRA). *Canadian ADHD Practice Guidelines, Third Edition*. CADDRA, 2011. https://caddra.ca/pdfs/caddraGuidelines2011.pdf.

Chandler, David L. "Study: Better sleep habits lead to better college grades." *MIT News*. October 1, 2019. https://news.mit.edu/2019/better-sleep-better-grades-1001.

Children and Adults with Attention-Deficit/Hyperactivity Disorder (CHADD). "General Prevalence of ADHD." CHADD.org. Accessed July 10, 2025. https://chadd.org/about-adhd/general-prevalence/.

Coghill, David R. "Organisation of services for managing ADHD." *Epidemiology and Psychiatric Science* 26, no. 5 (2016): 453–458. https://doi.org/10.1017/S2045796016000937.

Dalsgaard, Søren, Søren Dinesen Østergaard, James F. Leckman, Preben Bo Mortensen, and Marianne Giørtz Pedersen. "Mortality in children, adolescents, and adults with attention deficit hyperactivity disorder: a nationwide cohort study." *The Lancet* 385, no. 9983 (2015): 2190–2196. https://doi.org/10.1016/S0140-6736(14)61684-6.

Dean, Ben. "Interview with Edward 'Ned' Hallowell, MD." MentorCoach. May 1, 2015. https://www.mentorcoach.com/positive-psychology-coaching/interviews/interview-edward-ned-hallowell-md/.

Dodson, William. "New Insights into Rejection Sensitive Dysphoria." *ADDitude Magazine*. Updated May 9, 2025.

https://www.additudemag.com/rejection-sensitive-dysphoria-adhd-emotional-dysregulation/.

Doshi, Jalpa A., Paul Hodgkins, Jennifer Kahle, et al. "Economic Impact of Childhood and Adult Attention-Deficit/Hyperactivity Disorder in the United States." *Journal of the American Academy of Child and Adolescent Psychiatry* 51, no. 10 (2012): 990–1002. https://doi.org/10.1016/j.jaac.2012.07.008.

Faraone, Stephen V. "An Overview of Attention Deficit Hyperactivity Disorder." The ADHD Evidence Project. (2022): 35–36; 40–41. https://www.adhdevidence.org/resources#slides.

Faraone, Stephen V., Tobias Banaschewski, David Coghill, Yi Zheng, Joseph Biederman, Mark A. Bellgrove. "The World Federation of ADHD International Consensus Statement: 208 Evidence-based conclusions about the disorder." *Neuroscience Biobehavior* 128 (2021): 789–818. https://doi.org/10.1016/j.neubiorev.2021.01.022.

Fava, Maurizio, Richard C. Shelton, and John M. Zajecka. "Evidence for the use of 1-methylfolate combined with antidepressants in MDD." *Journal of Clinical Psychiatry* 82, no. 8 (2011): e25. https://pubmed.ncbi.nlm.nih.gov/21899813/.

Ford, Tamsin. "Transitional care for young adults with ADHD: transforming potential upheaval into smooth progression." *Epidemiology and Psychiatric Science* 29 (2020): e87. https://doi.org/10.1017/S2045796019000817.

Greenblatt, James. *Finally Focused: The Breakthrough Natural Treatment Plan for ADHD that Restores Attention, Minimizes Hyperactivity, and Helps Eliminate Drug Side Effects*. Harmony Press, 2017.

Grimm, Oliver, Thorsten M. Kranz, and Andreas Reif. "Genetics of ADHD: What Should the Clinician Know?" *Current Psychiatry Report* 22, no. 18 (2020). https://doi.org/10.1007/s11920-020-1141-x.

Hall, Charlotte L., Karen Newell, John Taylor, Kapil Sayal, Katie
    D. Swift, and Chris Hollis. "'Mind the gap'—mapping services
    for young people with ADHD transitioning from child to adult
    mental health services." *BMC Psychiatry* 13, no. 186 (2013): 186.
    https://doi.org/10.1186/1471-244X-13-186.

Hallowell, Edward and John Ratey. "ADHD Needs a Better Name.
    We Have One." *ADDitude Magazine*. Updated March 24, 2025.
    https://www.additudemag.com/attention-deficit-disorder-vast/.

Hilton, Michael F., Paul A. Scuffham, Judith E, Sheridan, Catherine
    M. Cleary, Nerina Vecchio, and Harvey A. Whiteford. "The Asso-
    ciation Between Mental Disorders and Productivity in Treated
    and Untreated Employees." *Journal of Occupational and Envi-
    ronmental Medicine* 51, no. 9 (2009): 996–1003. https://doi.
    org/10.1097/JOM.0b013e3181b2ea30.

Hinshaw, Stephen. "Girls and Women with ADHD" (webinar). *ADDi-
    tude* Magazine. October 16, 2018. https://www.youtube.com/
    watch?v=5y6W9C4rJXw.

Institute for Functional Medicine. "Functional Medicine Restores
    Healthy Function by Treating the Root Causes of Disease."
    IFM.org. Accessed June 19, 2025. https://www.ifm.org/
    functional-medicine. Used with permission.

The Institute for Functional Medicine. "Functional Medicine." IMF.
    org. Accessed June 5, 2025. https://www.ifm.org/.

Jellinek, Michael S. "Don't Let ADHD Crush Children's Self-Esteem."
    Clinical Psychiatry News, 38 (2010). https://www.thefreeli-
    brary.com/Don%27t+let+ADHD+crush+children%27s+self-
    esteem.-a0228519256.

Job Accommodation Network. JAN.org. Accessed June 5, 2025.
    https://askjan.org/.

Kane, Megan. "CYP2D6 Overview: Allele and Phenotype Frequen-
    cies." *Medical Genetics Summaries*. Victoria M. Pratt, Stuart A.
    Scott, Munir Pirmohamed, Bernard Esquivel, Brandi Kattman,

Adriana J. Malheiro, ed. 2021; rev. 2025. https://www.ncbi.nlm.nih.gov/books/NBK574601/.

Kuriyan, Aparajita B., William E. Pelham, Jr., and Brooke S. G. Molina. "Young Adult Educational and Vocational Outcomes of Children Diagnosed with ADHD." *Journal of Abnormal Child Psychology*, 41, no. 1 (2012): 27–41. https://doi.org/10.1007/s10802-012-9658-z.

Matheson, Lauren, Philip Asherson, Ian Chi Kei Wong, et al. "Adult ADHD patient experiences of impairment, service provision and clinical management in England: a qualitative study." *BMC Health Services Research* 13, no. 184 (2013). https://doi.org/10.1186/1472-6963-13-184.

McCabe, Jessica. *How to ADHD: An Insider's Guide to Working with Your Brain (Not Against It)*. Penguin Random House, 2024.

Mehren, Aylin, Markus Reichert, David Coghill, Helge H. O. Müller, Niclas Braun and Alexandra Philipsen. "Physical exercise in attention deficit hyperactivity disorder—evidence and implications for the treatment of borderline personality disorder." *Borderline Personality Disorder and Emotion Dysregulation* 7, no. 1 (2020). https://doi.org/10.1186/s40479-019-0115-2.

Miller, Alan L. "The methylation, neurotransmitter, and antioxidant connections between folate and depression." *Alternative Medicine Review* 13, no. 3 (2008): 216–226. https://pubmed.ncbi.nlm.nih.gov/18950248/.

Montano, C. Brendan and Joel Young. "Discontinuity in the Transition from Pediatric to Adult Health Care for Patients with Attention-Deficit/Hyperactivity Disorder." *Postgraduate Medicine* 124, no. 5 (2012): 23–32. https://doi.org/10.3810/pgm.2012.09.2591.

MTA Cooperative Group. "A 14-Month Randomized Clinical Trial of Treatment Strategies for Attention-Deficit/Hyperactivity

Disorder." *Archives of General Psychiatry—JAMA Psychiatry* 56, no. 12 (1999): 1073–1086. https://doi.org/10.1001/archpsyc.56.12.1073.

Muld, Berit Bihlar, Jussi Jokinen, Sven Bölte, and Tatja Hirvikoski. "Long-Term Outcomes of Pharmacologically Treated Versus Non-Treated Adults with ADHD and Substance Use Disorder: A Naturalistic Study." *Journal of Substance Abuse Treatment* 51 (2015): 82–90. https://doi.org/10.1016/j.jsat.2014.11.005.

Muriel, Clara. "90 Famous People with ADHD: Struggles & Strengths." Very Special Tales.com. Updated December 21, 2023. https://veryspecialtales.com/famous-people-with-adhd/.

National Institute for Health and Care Excellence (NICE). "Attention deficit hyperactivity disorder: diagnosis and management." *NICE Guideline NG87.* Updated 2019. https://www.nice.org.uk/guidance/ng87.

Pérez Ortega, Rodrigo. "Under-diagnosed and under-treated, girls with ADHD face distinct risks." *Knowable Magazine.* 2020. https://knowablemagazine.org/article/mind/2020/adhd-in-girls-and-women.

Psychological Testing Online. "Adult ADHD Self-Report Screening Scale, ASRS-5." Psytests.org. Accessed July 14, 2025. https://psytests.org/diag/asrs5en-run.html.

Quinn, Patricia, and Theresa Maitland. *On Your Own, A College Readiness Guide for Teens with ADHD/LD.* Magination Press, 2011.

Riggs, Paula, Theresa Winhusen, Robert D. Davies, et al. "Randomized Controlled Trial of Osmotic-Release Methylphenidate With Cognitive-Behavioral Therapy in Adolescents With Attention-Deficit/Hyperactivity Disorder and Substance Use Disorders." *Journal of the American Academy of Child & Adolescent Psychiatry* 50, no. 9 (2011): 903–914. https://doi.org/10.1016/j.jaac.2011.06.010.

Rosenberg, Marshall B. *Nonviolent Communications: A Language of Life: Life-Changing Tools for Healthy Relationships.* PuddleDancer, 2015.

Schlamadiner, Diana. "What Research Says About HRT and Breast Cancer Risk." Breast Cancer Research Foundation. 2024. https://www.bcrf.org/about-breast-cancer/hrt-breast-cancer-risk/.

Sehinson, Claire. "An Introduction to Neurodiversity in Clinical Practice." PsychiatryRedefined.org. 2023. https://www.psychiatryredefined.org/wp-content/uploads/2023/09/Claire-Sehinson-Introduction-to-Neurodiversity-in-Clinical-Practice_Psychiatry-Redefined.pdf.

Shah, Priya Florence. "21 Famous Neurodivergent People in History and Today." Blog Brandz.com (2024). https://www.blogbrandz.com/tips/famous-neurodivergent-people/#content.

Talha, Md, and Abdulla al Mahmud. Abstract: *Individualism and Family Breakdown: Examining cultural variation.* Preprint. 2024. https://www.researchgate.net/publication/380366252_Individualism_and_Family_breakdown_examining_cultural_variation.

TOVA, "The Test of Variables of Attention," TOVAtest.com. Accessed July 15, 2025. https://tovatest.com/.

Tsai, S. J. "Top 17 Famous Scientists With ADHD That You May Not Know." Sci Journal.org. Updated April 18, 2024. https://www.scijournal.org/articles/famous-scientists-with-adhd.

U.S. Centers for Disease Control and Prevention. "About Attention-Deficit/Hyperactivity Disorder (ADHD)." CDC.gov. 2024. https://www.cdc.gov/adhd/about/index.html.

U.S. Centers for Disease Control and Prevention. "Data and Statistics on ADHD." CDC.gov. 2024. https://www.cdc.gov/adhd/data/index.html.

U.S. Department of Education. "Frequently Asked Questions: Section 504 Free Appropriate Public Education (FAPE)." Laws and Policy. Updated January 13, 2025. https://www.ed.gov/laws-and-policy/civil-rights-laws/disability-discrimination/frequently-asked-questions-section-504-free-appropriate-public-education-fape.

U.S. Department of Justice. Civil Rights Division. "Introduction to the Americans with Disabilities Act." ADA.gov. Accessed July 2025. https://www.ada.gov/topics/intro-to-ada/.

Walker, Linda. "Should You Disclose Your ADHD at Work? Survey Says . . ." ADDA.org. 2016. https://adhdatwork.add.org/should-you-disclose-your-adhd-at-work-survey-says/.

Wallance, Jamina, Elroy Boers, Julien Ouellet, Mohammad H. Afzali and Patricia Conrod. "Screen time, impulsivity, neuropsychological functions and their relationship to growth in adolescent attention-deficit/hyperactivity disorder symptoms." *Scientific Reports* 13, no. 18108 (2023). https://doi.org/10.1038/s41598-023-44105-7.

WikiGrewal. "33 Celebrities Who've Opened Up About Having ADHD." WikiGrewal.com. Accessed August 4, 2025. https://www.wikigrewal.com/famous-people-who-have-adhd/.

Wilens, Timothy E. and Himanshu P. Upadhyaya, "Impact of substance use disorder on ADHD and its treatment." *Journal of Clinical Psychiatry* 68, no. 8 (2007): e20. https://pubmed.ncbi.nlm.nih.gov/17876905/

Zhang, Le, Honghui Yao, Lin Li, et al., "Risk of Cardiovascular Diseases Associated With Medications Used in Attention-Deficit/Hyperactivity Disorder: A Systematic Review and Meta-analysis," *JAMA Network Open* 5, no. 11 (2022): e2243597. https://doi.org/10.1001/jamanetworkopen.2022.43597.

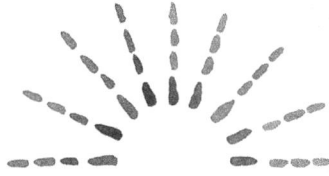

About the Author

Maggie Alexander's drive to educate the public and fellow clinicians about ADHD reflects her own transformation. When her children were still teens and she joked that she thought broccoli, love, and exercise could address most mental health challenges, she did not believe in ADHD. A single client opened her mind to its existence and propelled her down a path that resulted in her becoming highly skilled in treating this misunderstood and unique brain presentation.

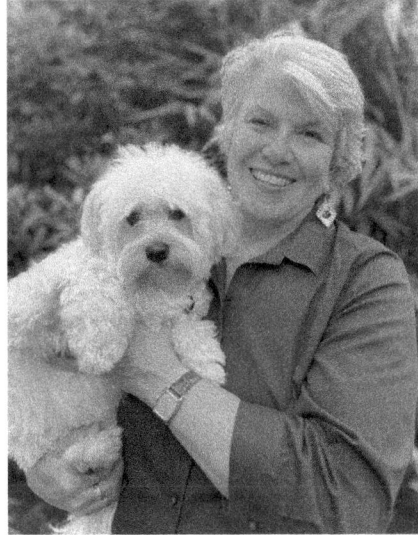

She delights in assisting individuals and families in discovering how to live happier, more productive lives. Whether consulting with a new client or seeing progress in the individuals she has seen develop over years, she is excited for their future.

Maggie is eager to conduct more seminars for providers around the country. She inspires hope by assisting one person, family, and community at a time. This is accomplished through the most current research and successful tools for transforming the lives of people with ADHD.

Before stepping into mental health care, Maggie attended to women and families as a certified nurse midwife. She has two master's degrees in nursing and has been an educator at Oregon Health & Science University. She is known for her kind and empowering style that honors the unique ways we all present, and she is actively increasing her focus on mentoring other clinicians. She lives in Portland, Oregon, where she enjoys her family, horseback riding, and walking in the forest with her dog.

Maggie's website will give you access to materials for the public to help you talk with your health professionals. If you are a clinician who is interested in applying these principles in your practice, consider inviting her to do a webinar or receiving individualized supervision.

shinewithadhdbook@gmail.com

maggiealexandernp.com

A portion of the sales of this book will go to offering treatment to individuals with ADHD who cannot afford care.

The B Corp Movement

Dear reader,

Thank you for reading this book and joining the Publish Your Purpose community! You are joining a special group of people who aim to make the world a better place.

What's Publish Your Purpose About?

Our mission is to elevate the voices often excluded from traditional publishing. We intentionally seek out authors and storytellers with diverse backgrounds, life experiences, and unique perspectives to publish books that will make an impact in the world.

Certified

(B)

Corporation

Beyond our books, we are focused on tangible, action-based change. As a woman- and LGBTQ+-owned company, we are committed to reducing inequality, lowering levels of poverty, creating a healthier environment, building stronger communities, and creating high-quality jobs with dignity and purpose.

As a Certified B Corporation, we use business as a force for good. We join a community of mission-driven companies building a more equitable, inclusive, and sustainable global economy. B Corporations must meet high standards of transparency, social and environmental performance, and accountability as determined by the nonprofit B Lab. The certification process is rigorous and ongoing (with a recertification requirement every three years).

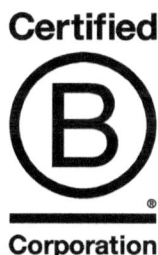

How Do We Do This?

We intentionally partner with socially and economically disadvantaged businesses that meet our sustainability goals. We embrace and encourage our authors and employee's differences in race, age, color, disability, ethnicity, family or marital status, gender identity or expression, language, national origin, physical and mental ability, political affiliation, religion, sexual orientation, socio-economic status, veteran status, and other characteristics that make them unique.

Community is at the heart of everything we do—from our writing and publishing programs to contributing to social enterprise nonprofits like reSET (https://www.resetco.org/) and our work in founding B Local Connecticut.

We are endlessly grateful to our authors, readers, and local community for being the driving force behind the equitable and sustainable world we are building together.

To connect with us online, or publish with us, visit us at www.publishyourpurpose.com.

Elevating Your Voice,

Jenn T Grace

Jenn T. Grace
Founder, Publish Your Purpose

www.ingramcontent.com/pod-product-compliance
Lightning Source LLC
Chambersburg PA
CBHW041157280326
41927CB00019BA/3377